EIGHT SHORT WEEKS TO A LIFETIME OF GOOD HEALTH

WEEK #1: With the h[...] tutes, you [...] and enjoy [...] and better [...]

WEEK #2: Following a step-by-step program that includes a vital supplement, you kick the *sugar* habit—and reduce your risks of contracting heart disease, diabetes, and other health problems.

WEEK #3: You add good *nutrition* to your life with regular meals, healthful shopping and snacking tips, and nutritional principles that improve your metabolism, digestion, and overall health.

WEEK #4: Your easiest week! You benefit from *vitamins and minerals* in supplement doses tailored for your age group, sex, and life-style.

WEEK #5: You eliminate the harmful effects of *alcohol*, as you find out how even moderate drinking impairs sexual performance, your gastrointestinal system, good nutrition, and more.

WEEK #6: You learn how to integrate *exercise* into your life with special tips on safety, setting realistic goals, and making exercise a real and enjoyable enhancement to your life.

WEEK #7: With a simple, four-point plan, you combat *stress* and discover what triggers tension in your life, learn a quick-fix stress reliever, and more!

WEEK #8: You stop *smoking* with the seven-day plan that psychologically and physically fights tobacco . . . and because it's part of the total *Medical Makeover* program, do it with little or, most likely, *no* permanent weight gain.

THE STARS COME OUT FOR

Medical

"He changed my life. He turned me around. He got me off caffeine, sugar, and salt. I think the world of him."
—Don Imus, *Radio Personality*, WNBC, New York

"Dr. Giller has his foot in the door of the future, yet he's a real doctor. I'm feeling great on his program."
—Blair Sabol, *Health Writer*

"My health is definitely better since I've been seeing Dr. Giller, and he has made me more aware of it."
—Len Cariou, *Actor*

"Dr. Giller is very skilled. He keeps everyone I know who goes to him in perfect health."
—Richard Ohrbach, *Interior Designer*

DR. GILLER AND HIS

Makeover

"I've sent dozens of friends and fellow workers to him. I'm a great believer in what he does."

—Bob O'Brien, *News Reporter*, Metromedia, New York

"The vitamins were of value and the exercise program he prescribed was of enormous benefit—both physically and mentally."

—Robert Summer, President, RCA Records

"He has really helped me with the stress and strain of performing every night. I just have terrific faith in him."

—Farley Granger, *Actor*

DR. GILLER has had a private practice in New York City since 1973. His patients include Liza Minnelli, Paul Simon, Bianca Jagger, George Hamilton, Nastassja Kinski, Mikhail Baryshnikov, Judy Collins, Natalia Makarova, and many other celebrities.

Medical Makeover

The Revolutionary No-Willpower Program for Lifetime Health

Robert M. Giller, M.D., and Kathy Matthews

WARNER BOOKS

A Warner Communications Company

WARNER BOOKS EDITION

This Warner Books Edition is published by arrangement with Beech Tree Books, William Morrow and Company, Inc., 105 Madison Avenue, New York, N.Y. 10016

Warner Books, Inc.
666 Fifth Avenue
New York, N.Y. 10103

A Warner Communications Company

Printed in the United States of America

First Warner Books Printing: June, 1987

10 9 8 7 6 5 4 3 2 1

To my patients,
who have helped me realize
that medicine is more
than a profession

Acknowledgments

To my parents, who encouraged good habits from the start; to Ruth Hoffman and Pete Kameron, who have become my family away from home; to my agent, Al Lowman, who encouraged me to write this book; and to my office manager, Judy Cramer, for her loyalty and support. And to Radu, for getting me into shape.

—R.M.G.

My deepest thanks to James Landis for his editorial vision and guidance; to Jane Meara, for her unflagging patience and unerring editorial judgment; and to Al Lowman, my much-prized agent, for making it all possible.

—K.M.

Contents

Part I: *THE CONCEPT*

Beyond Willpower 3
The Promise of Positive Medicine 21
Easing into the Makeover 34

Part II: *THE PROGRAM*

Week One: Caffeine 49
Week Two: Sugar 77
Week Three: The New Nutrition 120
Week Four: Vitamins and Minerals, the New
            Nutrition Supplements 156
Week Five: Alcohol 197
Week Six: Exercise 224
Week Seven: Stress Control 253
Week Eight: Smoking 278

Your Madeover Future 299

Sources 308

Index 316

PART I

THE CONCEPT

Beyond Willpower

When Jack L. first came to see me he seemed like the last person you would find waiting anxiously in a doctor's waiting room. There was, after all, nothing really wrong with him. In his mid-thirties, he would no doubt be considered a healthy man in the prime of life. But Jack was facing some big changes in his life, and he was worried that some minor symptoms he suffered from would become worse and he simply couldn't afford to have that happen.

Jack had just begun a demanding job in a new company with increased responsibilities. He had also just separated from his wife and moved into an apartment in the city. He was visiting his children as often as he could and keeping up with the social demands of his work, but he was beginning to feel worn out. He often had afternoon headaches. He knew he needed to lose some weight. He hadn't exercised, really exercised, since college when a wrestling injury had given him a chronic weakness and regular stiffness in his neck and shoulder. Jack was also finding that the entertaining he had to do in connection with his job meant that he was drinking

3

more than he would have liked. He was having up to six cups of coffee a day, just to keep going. He was starting to feel run down, and he knew he couldn't continue at the pace he had set if he weren't in optimum health.

Jack was at a turning point. His fast-paced life-style was encouraging bad health habits, and he knew that if he kept them up, his health would suffer and he wouldn't be able to handle his responsibilities. He was at the point where his habits were about to turn into addictions. I use the word "addictions" advisedly because that's precisely what our bad health habits become when they are repeated over a period of time. Jack, however, had not yet turned that corner.

Jack represents a new and very welcome kind of patient. He knows that if he ignores his health and lives with stress, a poor diet, no exercise, and too much drinking, he'll feel their effects, and his personal sense of well-being, as well as his ability to achieve success at work, will suffer. Jack knew all this, and so my job was almost half done. He just needed to know *how* to begin a program that would eliminate his bad habits and replace them with good ones. He needed more than a list of things to do and not to do; he needed an intelligent, effective method for accomplishing his goals.

Today Jack says that he feels ten years younger. He has more stamina than he would have thought possible. He's lost weight, and the combination of the exercise program he's adopted and the weight loss have given him almost complete relief from his nagging shoulder pain. His afternoon headaches are gone. He's able to eat out with his clients and not damage his health. He's handling the demands of his new job with more energy than he had when he first started with the position. His personal life is unresolved, but Jack says that just feeling in the peak of health makes him feel optimistic and in control of his future.

* * *

Kate S. is blond, attractive, articulate, and clearly intelligent. At twenty-eight years of age, Kate is a transplanted Texan living on the Upper West Side and working as an adjunct professor at the Columbia Graduate School of Journalism. She has worked at television stations in Dallas, Washington, and New York, and she has the kind of focus and determination that spell success. Speaking with her today it's hard to believe that a few months ago, in the middle of a well-prepared lecture to a class of graduate students, she felt so tired and unable to concentrate that she couldn't continue. She had been feeling sluggish and tired for a few weeks. But who doesn't occasionally feel tired, especially when they work at a driving pace? Certainly occasional fatigue was nothing to investigate. But now her sluggishness was beginning to interfere with her job.

When Kate came to see me she told me she didn't think that she was sick, but she certainly wasn't what she considered well. In fact, she mentioned that her symptoms sounded like depression, and she wanted to make it clear that in fact she was feeling very satisfied with her life. She loved her work, and the new course she was teaching at Columbia Graduate School of Journalism was a challenge. But she mentioned that she was not taking good care of her physical self. She was not exercising regularly. She ate what she considered were typical foods on a typical schedule, but she admitted that her meals were erratic. Kate could no longer ignore her symptoms. She had headaches a few times a week. She slept a lot but always felt tired. She had no energy or enthusiasm for anything. But the thing that frightened her the most was the problem she had concentrating. When she found herself faltering during a lecture, she knew something had to be done. Kate came to see me because she didn't want to take drugs for her headaches. She had heard from a friend that I would probably take a different approach to treating her.

When I questioned Kate, she revealed that in the last few months she had felt an increased need to smoke and was up to two packs a day. Because coffee was always available at her office, she had begun drinking more and more. She was drinking as many as four or five cups a day and had been for months. She craved sweets frequently, particularly the week or so before her period.

Unlike Jack's bad habits, Kate's had gone on for so long that they had become real addictions, and she craved cigarettes, coffee, and candy bars when she didn't have them. She craved them because they gave her a quick "fix" and she temporarily felt better. But Kate's highs no longer compensated for her frequent and troubling lows.

Now Kate says that she has far more energy and stamina than ever before. She has lost weight even though she says that she feels like she is eating constantly. She sleeps less and better. The last time I saw her, she told me that her friends say they see a difference in her and they even hear it in her voice. She says that she feels as if she's living a whole different, better life.

Tom G. works on one of the highest floors of the World Trade Center in downtown Manhattan, and his fight to become well was no less dramatic than the view from the windows of his office. Slim and erect at forty years of age, Tom has a robust appearance today that belies the man who came to see me two years ago.

Tom had been doing his best to ignore all the warning signals that should have alerted him to his dangerous situation. He was feeling run down and under tremendous pressure from a failing business and a bitter child custody battle with his ex-wife: His health, he figured, would just have to take a backseat until he got his life in order. He was addicted to cigarettes—two and a half packs a day—and sweet, black coffee. He never exercised and ate mostly junk food—greasy take-out hamburgers, fried chicken, and pizza. He wasn't fat, but in the past year his weight was climbing upward. "I was either smoking, eating, drinking coffee, or sleeping," he says of that difficult time.

At age thirty-eight, it all caught up with him: He had a heart attack.

He says it took him by surprise since he was such a young man. And, in fact, it made a new man of him. He would never have listened to warnings about his health. He needed a life-threatening scare to force him to make changes. When Tom came to see me, he was frightened.

Today Tom regards his old devil-may-care attitude toward his health with disgust. He can hardly believe that he could have continued to endanger his life so thoughtlessly and even knowingly. Because Tom knew that someday he might have to pay a price for his life-style. He just kept thinking that "someday" was way off in the future.

Tom still has problems: His business eventually did fail, and he lost the custody battle with his wife. His new job as a commodity trader is very pressured. But Tom feels more capable of handling his troubles. As he says, "I don't know if my life is less stressful today or if I'm simply better able to handle things. Either way, my life is on track again and I feel optimistic and energetic. In fact, my energy level is higher than it's ever been. In retrospect, that heart attack was a blessing in disguise. If I'd had it when I was older, I might not be here today. And it forced me to change my life. The new me is really a happier and more successful person."

Jack, Kate, and Tom's transformations are typical of the changes I've witnessed in patients who have been coming to see me over the past ten years. These people initially came to me because I have a reputation as a doctor who is reluctant to rely on drugs as the only remedy for health problems. These patients are what I've come to call "medical makeovers": people who have dramatically changed their lives, their health, their sense of well-being, and possibly their longevity by following a step-by-step program that I call the Medical Makeover.

The Medical Makeover in Capsule

The Medical Makeover you're going to read about in this book is unlike any other diet or self-improvement program you've ever heard about. It's a brand-new—I'll even go so far as to say revolutionary—approach to health care that will make you feel as healthy and energetic as you did when you were a kid. Maybe even better. It tackles the major factors affecting your health and well-being, using a system that has proven effective with the thousands of patients I've been able to help.

Depending on your health habits, the Makeover takes eight weeks or less, and each week of the program is devoted to a specific area of health improvement, guiding you to break bad habits and find your optimum health life-style.

Optimum health is an interrelationship that depends on the orchestration of many factors. The Medical Makeover takes into account the fact that *any single fitness, nutrition, or stress-management program that is undertaken in isolation is ultimately doomed to failure*.

The Medical Makeover has both short- and long-term effects. The short-term effect is to make you feel great today. The long-term effect is to help you beat the odds against developing a chronic, killing disease in the future. The medical research breakthroughs that make these two goals achievable exist, but they have never before been put into a simple, effective program that takes into account the physical and psychological difficulties of making changes in your life. The Medical Makeover will be your blueprint to a healthy life-style, today and in the years to come.

Are You a Victim of Vague Symptoms?

I believe that vague symptoms are the plague of modern living. I couldn't begin to count the patients who have come to my office over the years suffering from minor but persistent problems. These people think of themselves as generally healthy, and they are mystified by their bodies' rebellion. An occasional headache is acceptable, they think, but they seem to get a headache several times a week. They expect to be tired at the end of the day, but, they ask, is it normal to be exhausted at four in the afternoon—so tired that you can fall asleep at your desk? And what about an inability to concentrate? So many patients tell me that they often find it almost impossible to set their minds to the task at hand. One patient of mine who was a copywriter told me that if she didn't get her copy done first thing in the morning it was a hopeless task; she was, as she put it, "worthless" in the afternoon. So many patients complain of feeling tired and irritable, and they eventually believe that only a super-human effort allows them to accomplish anything at all.

Unfortunately, many people assume that these vague symptoms are an inevitable part of aging and stress. They see the body as a machine with a limited useful span. They figure by the time they're past twenty or thirty or forty years old, they're beginning to run down and have to expect and accept the aches and pains and fatigue of an "older machine." Well, the human life span is certainly limited, but the vital, energetic period we are given to enjoy our bodies is limited *only* by our approach to health care. Many of the discomforts and maladies we ascribe to age or stress are avoidable.

If, like most people, you dismiss vague symptoms as an inevitable part of your life, you should know that the most pernicious aspect of the most common killers in our country—coronary heart disease and cancer—is that they creep up on their victims gradually and slowly, sometimes over a period of many years. And early symptoms of future disability—headaches, afternoon fatigue, inability to concentrate, sleeplessness, depression, susceptibility to colds—are all warning signals that are too easily dismissed. You do not simply wake up one day with cancer or heart disease; *it takes years of bad habits and minor symptoms before you find yourself facing serious disease*. Even as you read this, your body may be trying to warn you of future chronic disease in some subtle way.

People are encouraged to ignore their vague symptoms. For one thing, it's assumed that there's no way to treat them; for another, it's assumed that they're not dangerous. And finally many people feel that they should "tough it out" when it comes to vague symptoms. The people who are sheepish about complaining of regular, if mild, health problems are the same ones who pride themselves on showing up at work unless they have to be hospitalized. They're so used to ignoring the signals their bodies are sending them that they're amazed to learn about the connection between their symptoms and their future health.

I believe that many of the mild symptoms that are thought of as psychosomatic may be real psychological warning signals that, if ignored, will develop into chronic disease. It has also been my experience that many patients with these early warning signs have been told by their physicians that their diagnostic tests are WNL (within normal limits) and that they are suffering from stress. Common solutions to these everyday medical mysteries include recommendations from friends, family, and doctors to relax, take a vacation, lose some weight, stop drinking, join a health club, or try another doctor. None of this advice tells you how to do these things, and worse, it may encourage you to neglect the early warning signs of serious illness and to spend years of your life in suboptimum health.

I Know I Should Change, but . . .

Would you like to feel good, really good, when you wake up in the morning? Would you like to have more energy for work and recreation? Would you like to look better, be slimmer and stronger? Would you like to be free of afternoon fatigue, headaches, irritability?

And what about your future . . . ? Would you like to live longer? Or, more to the point, would you like to be healthier for more years of your life and have a vital, active old age?

Absurd questions, you may think, but even as you answer "of course" to all of them, you may be contradicting yourself. Did you have a cup of coffee this morning and a few more during the day? Did you skip breakfast? Do you smoke? Are you overweight? Have you been drinking a bit more than you feel you should? Do you have a regular exercise program? What about the stress in your life: Are you doing something to counteract it?

These questions about your life-style really say more about how you feel now and will feel in the future than any assertions you may make to the contrary. *If you don't live well, you don't feel well—now or in the future. Your habits determine your health.* The Medical Makeover is based on that simple, proven fact. But it takes that fact one step further. The Medical Makeover uses a revolutionary technique to help you *change* and *improve* your habits so that you can be healthy now and in the future. Once you understand how your mind and your body shape your habits and how you need to work with both to change them, you'll see why the Medical Makeover will work even if other programs have failed you.

If you've ever begun a diet but failed, tried to begin an exercise program but abandoned it after a short time, stopped smoking a few dozen times, or tried to cut down on your coffee intake but found it not worth the effort, you are painfully aware that just knowing the facts about life-style and disease doesn't really help you to change your behavior. Knowing you should do something isn't enough to help you meet your goal. Behavioral medicine is the new science that gives us the hard evidence that our life-style affects our health. Unfortunately, it doesn't help us *change* our lives. And that, of course, is the crux of the problem.

Most of the basic tenets of healthy living have been known for years. We've heard them from our mothers and grandmothers from the time we were small children. We are all aware of how important it is to eat right, exercise, stop smoking, get plenty of rest, and so forth. Maybe most of us don't know that the three main causes of death in this country are preventable. But even if we knew that and also how to avoid these threats, would we do so? Certainly my own personal experience, and that of my patients, argue that we wouldn't. The simple fact is that most of us have no real comprehensive approach to keeping ourselves healthy. Why not? Because it really doesn't seem to matter in any immediate, tangible way. Sure, we've all been on blitz diets or short-lived exercise programs. Often we make sporadic efforts to take care of ourselves after a scare—a personal confrontation with serious illness or death—or a temporary high, like the good feeling that accompanies a few weeks of exercise. But then things go back to business as usual.

There's a bit of the gambler in us all. When you read about a ninety-year-old man who smokes a pack of cigarettes a day and drinks a quart of corn whiskey a week, do you feel relieved? "Whew! It works for him; it just might work for me. And besides, I don't smoke quite that much."

I used to be like that. Our culture encourages us to live hard, ignore the obvious, and hope for the best. In 1976 the tobacco industry spent $400 million on advertising. The government spent $2.2 million to educate us to the dangers of smoking cigarettes. If you want to gamble with your health, you have lots of expensive encouragement.

We're also chained to the status quo by a conservatism in the scientific community that would have each link of the chain firmly in place before action is recommended. At least five years before the Surgeon General's 1964 report officially proclaimed cigarettes were a hazard, there was sufficient evidence to issue a warning to smokers. Nathan Pritikin's low-fat diet was scoffed at by scientists for many years, and is only now being accepted as a valuable approach to preventing cardiovascular disease. Naturally there is a sound basis for caution in regard to medical recommendations, but you really can't afford to wait until everyone is in agreement on such basic matters as healthy diet and the dangers of sugar, caffeine, alcohol, stress, and cigarettes.

There are so many reasons to continue as we are and, worse yet, tell ourselves that the one or two things we do to try to become healthy are enough. Most of us have developed our own inconsistent health "rules" that we follow but are not really making an appreciable difference in the way we feel because other bad habits sabotage their good effects. Perhaps you avoid fats but drink several cups of coffee every day. Perhaps you exercise regularly, but your diet is hit or miss and you don't believe vitamins make much of a difference. Perhaps you gave up smoking but get no regular exercise. Perhaps you think that drinking every night, as long as you never become inebriated, doesn't make much difference and is something you deserve, something that is crucial to your enjoyment of life.

Or perhaps you subscribe to the "checks and balances" system of health care: drink too much but take vitamins to compensate; live with killing stress but make a point of never eating sweets. If you do, you're not alone. Studies have shown that many people live by this system. People who exercise often feel that it will compensate for their poor diet.

Most of us simply don't have enough motivation to change our regular habits—all our bad habits—in a way that would truly affect our health every single day of our lives. We cling to them because we see them as rewards for a hard day at the office or a difficult task accomplished or a trying morning at the dentist.

It's this enormous resistance to change that we must overcome if we want to achieve optimum health.

When I began to see the patients described in the beginning of this book, they had one thing in common: They all knew that they were probably going to have to make some changes in behavior in order to feel better. They had been to other doctors. They had had all the routine tests done, and the tests had all been negative. They had tried all the medications. They had come to me because a friend or colleague or another doctor had suggested that I might be able to help. Most of them knew that I specialized in nutrition, and they expected, at the very least, to change their diet. They wanted to make changes. They were prepared to do what I suggested. They were paying me to tell them exactly how to change their lives so they would feel better. But despite how poorly they felt, how much they wanted to change, how eager they were to follow my suggestions, the simple fact was that when it actually came down to making changes in their habits, very, very few of them were successful.

This failure was a mystery to me, and it was what inspired me to begin the work that resulted in the

Medical Makeover. Now I know that my patients were typical. The depressing fact is that education alone is not enough. In fact, a study done in 1978 by Louis Harris only confirms what I was seeing in my patients. Most Americans have unhealthy habits and live unhealthy lives and they know it but *can't* change. Fully 67 percent recognize that they would be healthier if they ate more of some foods and less of others. And fully 70 percent of smokers know that their habit increases their chances of getting cancer, and yet they still smoke. Two out of every five Americans believe that they ought to exercise more than they do. Two out of every three think they would be healthier if they changed their diets, but they continue to eat the way they do because they enjoy their unhealthy diets and lack the willpower to change.

Curiously enough, this poll also revealed that out of the eight goals that people consider important, including peace of mind, having close friends, and getting and keeping a good job, the overwhelming majority—70 percent—put good health at the top of the list.

So there you have it. We know we should change but we can't. You know you should change, and that's why you are reading this book. You may need convincing in some areas—for example, you may think that drinking coffee is not bad for you, but I have plenty of evidence to convince you that you're wrong. I'm sure that as far as exercise, diet, smoking, and drinking are concerned, you know that you could use improvement. You just need to know how to do it in a way that will really work for you.

Why the Medical Makeover Will Work for You, or Beyond Willpower

The secret to success in any kind of behavioral change has always been identified as "willpower." In the Harris poll mentioned above, the reason for people's failure to change in the face of overwhelming evidence that they should is given as "lack of willpower." You probably think that the reason you have fallen off diets or exercise programs in the past is your own lack of willpower. I think that willpower is only part of the story.

One of the problems with depending on willpower is that it makes success a *moral* issue. If you have the strength of character, the willpower, to stick to a program, you're a good person. If you don't, if you have a piece of chocolate cake or a cigarette, or if you skip exercise class, then you are by definition a failure. That's quite a burden to carry around. It makes the whole issue of diet or exercise distasteful; no one likes to do something that makes them feel like a failure. Finally if you do fail, you're worse off than before you started because you're more reluctant than ever to try to change. One of my patients, before she successfully completed the Makeover, was a perfect example of this self-improvement backlash. As she said, "I've learned something about myself in the past few years after all the diet and exercise programs I've been on: I can do anything, absolutely anything, for two weeks. But I can't stick with the simplest program for three."

There's no question you can't make changes without the determination to change—and that, in a sense, is willpower. But it will only get you started. To stick to a program of change you need more than the decision to do so. You need to know how to go about making the changes and how to make your **body** work for you as you change. The Medical Makeover is the first program that takes both these elements into consideration, and that's why it's so successful.

Even if you've failed to improve your habits in the past, I think you'll succeed with the Medical Makeover. Because this program takes a proven, double-barreled approach to behavioral change. To improve your habits you need both *psychological* and *physiological* techniques.

The Medical Makeover is unique in providing both. In fact, the Medical Makeover is built on the combination of two breakthroughs: one psychological, one physiological.

The *psychological* approach takes habits seriously. This is the first popular book to adopt a program of habit change that treats habits as addictions. You need all the help to break your habits that a hard-core addict needs to kick heroin, because these habits are tightly woven into the fabric of your life. Any program that doesn't acknowledge that fact is doomed to failure.

For example, you began to have coffee in the morning over a period of time. Perhaps at one point you started having a Danish with the coffee. Soon it became an established ritual: You would stop at the coffee shop on the way to work. The guy behind the counter knows you. You greet each other, share a few pleasantries, and he wraps up your order. Just carrying it into your office feels good. You're eager to take that first sip of coffee and taste the great sweetness of that Danish. The whole experience is really very satisfying. To change your routine—to stop having coffee, give up the Danish—without considering how much this habit means to you is too much to ask. If you do give up your habit, but not in a methodical, systematic way that takes into account what that habit means to you, it probably won't be for long. Habits are hard to break and you need psychological help to give them up.

The *physiological* approach recognizes that many of your bad habits are **biochemically** determined. To break them you need to change your metabolism. You need to make your body an ally rather than an enemy.

You develop bad habits because they feel good. They feel good because they have an effect on the body that is pleasurable or useful or both. Drinking that morning coffee and eating that Danish have a similar effect: They raise your blood sugar and give you a boost of energy. If you give up coffee and Danish, you're going to feel terrible because you'll miss the wonderful jolt you depended on to get you started in your day. But if you compensate for that jolt, or get it some other way so that you don't feel let down and tired, you're going to find it easier to give up coffee and Danish. That's what the Medical Makeover will do for you. With the modification of diet, the use of vitamin and mineral supplements, and the substitution of new habits, it will help you adjust your body chemistry so that it won't be fighting the changes you're making.

I've had many patients who craved sweets and never imagined they could give them up. Mary G., a television scriptwriter, was in the habit of having a sweet roll in the morning, sometimes a candy bar in the middle of the day, and dessert with lunch. In addition, she drank three or four cups of coffee per day with two teaspoons of sugar in each. Mary was willing to make the effort to give up sugar, but she really didn't believe that she could. She carefully worked out ways to change her coffee and sweets habits, but she anticipated she would feel deprived at best. Mary was astonished to find that a mineral—chromium—really affected her desire for sweets.

Chromium is the supplement you'll be taking to help control the highs and lows of blood sugar that make you feel tired and irritable. This is an example of how the Medical Makeover can help your body become an ally instead of any enemy. By taking chromium Mary was successful at controlling her sweet tooth; she was very pleased at the change in her moods and energy level and in the weight loss that resulted because she reduced her daily calorie intake. I'm certain that if Mary had depended on just her willpower to stay away from sweets, the task would have been formidable. But with the help of chromium to stabilize her metabolism, giving up sugar wasn't such a terrible ordeal.

This combination of the psychological and physiological approaches is revolutionary, and I think it will be the help you need to change your life and health for the better. It's a sort of built-in motivation. The changes will be easier to make than you think because your metabolism will be altered. And the program will be easier to stick with because the motivation will come from your own body. You'll feel so noticeably better that you'll want to continue. By the end of your eight weeks, the Medical Makeover will no longer be a program—it will be your new "health style."

Are You Ready for a Medical Makeover?

If you think of yourself as healthy, but you suffer from:

- frequent headaches
- afternoon fatigue
- insomnia
- overweight
- frequent colds, sore throats, and other infections
- irritability
- digestive problems

you could be a candidate for a Medical Makeover.

If you think of yourself as healthy and you:

- exercise but sometimes skip breakfast
- never skip breakfast but have coffee and a sweet in the afternoon as a pick-me-up
- limit your caffeine and alcohol but rarely exercise
- exercise regularly but eat sporadically
- eat what you consider a good healthy diet but don't take any vitamin supplements
- take vitamins regularly but smoke

• don't smoke but sleep fewer than seven hours per night

you could be a candidate for a Medical Makeover—a change in your health habits that will affect the way you feel each and every day, now and for the rest of your life.

The Promise of
Positive Medicine

Chosen Illnesses

We're not as healthy as we think we are. Although most Americans are convinced that with sophisticated medical techniques and wide public awareness of health issues they're getting healthier and healthier, it depends on how you look at it. While it's true, according to the U.S. Census Bureau, that our death rate is dropping, it's also true that our disability rate is climbing. The National Institute on Aging, a division of the National Institutes of Health, says that rates of illness, particularly chronic illness, are increasing most rapidly among the group aged forty-five to sixty-four. By age sixty-five most people have well-established ailments. Today for a man of forty-five, life expectancy is only five years greater than it was in 1900. So we may be around longer, but those extra years are plagued by poor health. Why? Because there's only so much that medical science can do to keep us from becoming ill; the rest is in our hands and we haven't been doing a very good job.

Taking into consideration the fact that we need help if

we're going to become healthier, there is a revolution going on in health care today. "Behavioral medicine" or "health promotion" are the terms most commonly given to describe this new approach, which is based on a simple if astounding fact: Over fifty percent of the mortality from the ten leading causes of death in this country today can be traced to life-style. Countless sophisticated studies have demonstrated a very simple cause and effect between life-style and your life span.

Nedra Belloc and Lester Breslow have done some of the pioneering work on habits and morbidity and mortality. After studying the lives of seven thousand men and women in California, they correlated both physical well-being and life span to adherence to seven basic practices:

1. Sleeping seven to eight hours each night
2. Eating three meals a day at regular hours with little snacking
3. Eating breakfast every day
4. Maintaining optimum body weight
5. Avoiding excessive alcohol consumption
6. Regular exercise
7. Not smoking

This may not sound like ground-breaking information to you, but it was "news" to the medical profession when it was published as recently as 1977. And consider the following: Belloc and Breslow found that people who adopted all seven basic habits were about as physically healthy as people thirty years younger who followed few or none of these habits. Even more specific, they stated that a man who is forty-five years old and who follows three or fewer of these habits will probably live to be sixty-seven. But a man who follows six or seven of the listed habits will probably live to be seventy-eight! *That's eleven extra years of life.*

How can this be? How can you live longer just by eating breakfast every day and exercising? Remember that the most common **killer** diseases today are chronic and degenerative. They are heart disease and cancer. These diseases are affected by life-style. **If you smoke, you increase your chances of developing cancer. If you eat a high-fat diet, you're more likely to develop heart disease.** You can think of these common killers as "chosen illnesses," because the decisions that you are making today about what you eat and how you live are determining whether or not you will develop one or more of these diseases.

Some simple statistics will show that developing a dread disease like cancer is not a matter of a "health lottery" or "genetic roulette," as some of us think. One third of the population will develop cancer in his or her lifetime. Cancer accounted for 21 percent of all deaths in 1984. But we could prevent most of these deaths with simple changes in our health habits because research has shown that 70 to 80 percent of all cancers are produced by diet or life-style choices, including smoking and drinking.

Given this information, you can see that your "bad habits" are really more serious than you might have thought. And in the ten years since the Belloc-Breslow study was published, other habits have been recognized as "bad." Yes, drinking coffee is a bad habit. But it also can contribute to heart disease in the future. And today it's probably wreaking havoc with how you feel by affecting your moods, your energy level, and your performance. (It's not the performance-enhancer you might think it is, and I'll tell you why in the chapter on caffeine.) Drinking alcohol is also a bad habit as are smoking and not exercising and eating an inadequate diet. All these bad habits, particularly in combination, are changing your life by causing vague symptoms today and sowing the seeds of future illness.

The Promise of Positive Medicine

I can't emphasize strongly enough that while your bad habits are setting you up for chronic illness in the future, they're also making you feel sick today.

Most of us feel pretty much the same each day. One day may be better or worse than the next, but our general condition remains the same. The little complaints we have may seem no more than minor ones to us. The simple fact is, we have grown so accustomed to feeling just OK that it never occurs to us that we could feel much, much better.

I tell my patients, and I am telling you, that you can expect to feel more vital and alive and that you will live longer once you've completed the Medical Makeover. I want you to have all the incentive possible to undertake it. You may think you feel just fine. I want you to know that you can feel much better. That's the promise of the Medical Makeover: You will live a healthier and happier life, not only in the near future, but in the here and now.

The Doctor's Dilemma

Did you know that the medical system in the United States—that is, doctors, drugs, and hospitals—can fairly take credit for only about *10 percent* of our collective health? The other 90 percent is due to our personal health habits—our life-styles.

Too great a belief on the part of the public, as well as the medical profession, in drugs and surgery as the solution to disease encourages people to persist in unhealthy life-styles and causes them to develop chronic diseases that are often beyond the abilities of modern medicine to vanquish completely. Television, of course, encourages instant cures. They can be wrapped up in a half hour, and once you're cured on TV, you're cured forever. You never have to worry about any follow-up or life-style change. Such beliefs are not only unrealistic and dangerous as far as our concept of health care is concerned, they also ignore the fact that drugs are not necessarily benign substances, and that they affect not just the problem or disease but the entire body and, as we learned from Valium, sometimes in tragic ways.

It is unrealistic and counterproductive to live by the "machine theory" of health, the belief that one can virtually run one's body into the ground by destructive health habits and then expect a doctor to come to the rescue at the last minute with a miracle drug or surgical procedure that will restore the body to good working order. *The cure for a chosen illness is prevention, and prevention is often a matter of changing life-style.*

Your doctor does not like to be frustrated. He wants to find out what's wrong with you and cure you. But he can't give you a prescription for a different way of life. His medical training didn't prepare him to teach you about nutrition and help you modify your habits. A dozen years ago when I was still in medical training the concept of preventive medicine in private practice didn't exist. Nutrition and diet were ignored. Most of the doctors' time in the hospital was spent with the 0.1 percent of sick patients who had chronic diseases, and we could only treat their symptoms.

Your doctor may already have told you to lose weight or stop smoking or cut down on your stress. He may explain the frightening statistics being published by researchers in behavioral medicine, but they don't help him convince you that you have to "clean up your act." I know how doctors feel in this situation because I've been there. I know how dismaying it is to have patients who don't feel well but have "nothing wrong with them," patients who are headed for chronic illness but can't change their habits.

The Medical Makeover is an effort to fill the wide gap

between the exciting discoveries of behavior medicine and the practical day-to-day changes you can make to improve the way you feel now and your longevity. The precepts of my program are simple, but the approach is unique. I think it could change your life.

The Origins of the Medical Makeover

When I set out to create the Makeover program, I soon realized that what I was doing was filling a gap. A great deal of up-to-the-minute medical information was available on how to improve your health. It appeared in all the medical journals, and many physicians were aware of it. But there was no translation of this material into practical terms, no way to use it to improve people's lives.

For example, many of my patients have problems with sugar. They go on sweet binges and have trouble sticking with a diet because as soon as they're faced with a doughnut or a box of candy, resolutions fly out the window. These patients have often become discouraged over the years, believing they could never stick to a weight-loss diet because they "had no willpower." They were victims of the "sweet tooth" myth. In fact, a sweet tooth is not something you're born with; it's the body's complex reaction to sugar that can create a vicious circle and drive you to sweet binges.

Many research projects have demonstrated that there is a trace mineral—chromium—that helps the body stabilize its use of sugar. I found that the patients taking chromium had little trouble keeping their cravings for sweets under control. They didn't need willpower, they needed actually to change their bodies' metabolisms, and chromium allowed them to do just that.

I found that being on the "front lines" and working with patients every day gave me the opportunity to use the latest research findings in a practical way for my own and my patients' benefit. The bottom line in developing the Medical Makeover has always been results. I simply used what worked and abandoned what didn't.

As I perfected the Medical Makeover, I enjoyed greater and greater success in helping my patients change their lives. A recent card from a young woman who lost over forty pounds on the Makeover program is typical: "I know this might sound crazy, but you have given me the best present I ever had. You gave me—me. It's not only a physical change though, it's a total change in my approach to life and it's very exciting. I'm a walking advertisement for you and all my friends want to try the Makeover. They call you my 'miracle worker.'" Responses like this made me realize that many, many people could benefit from my program, and that's why I decided to write this book.

I think of the Medical Makeover as an invitation and a challenge. I believe it will really change your life.

The Medical Makeover Breakthroughs: Why This Book Will Help You Where Others Have Failed

The Medical Makeover really works. It works because it's different. It incorporates the very latest medical research in a simple and practical program. It has six breakthroughs that make it different from every other program you might have tried or read about:

A Step-by-Step, Week-by-Week Approach

The Medical Makeover plans your time for you and tells you precisely what health habit you will be working on each week. It takes a simple, progressive approach that's very easy to follow. In the past you may have tried to change your life overnight and have failed. With the Medical Makeover, you won't try to change your life overnight: You'll proceed gradually, building success on success.

Each week of the Makeover builds on the prior week, reinforcing the good habits you've already learned and giving you the confidence to continue. Maryanne D., an advertising copywriter, said recently after completing the Makeover, "If anyone had told me going into this that I would be able to make all these changes I would have told them, 'You're crazy.' I just didn't think I had the capacity to stick with it. But doing it a few steps at a time made the difference. I never could have done it any other way."

Built-in Motivation

The motivation to continue the Medical Makeover will come from your own body. You will begin to feel better a few days into the first week. My patients have all said that they are amazed at how quickly they see results from following the program. When you begin to see change, when you begin to feel better and have more energy, it will give you the motivation to continue. As one patient told me, "Now I know how it feels to feel bad and how it feels to feel good. That makes it easy to stick with the program. I don't want to give up feeling as good as I do now."

Comprehensive Change

The bad habits that we have were developed over the years. I've noticed that one bad habit leads to another. Additionally, whenever we are under stress, we're inclined to depend on our bad habits even more: We have another cup of coffee, have that sweet we've been denying ourselves, have that extra cigarette or drink.

To be truly healthy, we must break the cycle, not just try to stop one bad habit and continue the others. Unless we deal with the total picture we're ultimately doomed to failure.

William F. is an advertising space salesman who came to me with chronic headaches. He had tried almost every medication and felt, as he said, "drugged out." After the Makeover, he no longer has headaches. Why? I think a combination of factors was causing them. As he says, "I now know that sugar was causing a problem. And so was my diet. It was so unvaried and not especially nutritious. Caffeine was a big item, maybe the major one. And stress management could have made the crucial difference. All I know now is that I'm not taking any drugs and I'm not having any headaches. We took every possible factor that could have been causing a problem and blitzed them one by one. Was it one particular problem or a combination of things that caused the headaches? To be honest, I don't know and I don't care. All I know is that they're gone and I feel great."

Effective Sequence

The eight-week sequence of the Medical Makeover has been carefully worked out to alter your body chemistry gradually and make it easier for you to stick to the new habits you'll be developing. No other health program has ever taken this biologically determined sequential approach. You'll find that following this sequence will make changes possible (if not easy) that you may have found impossible to achieve in the past.

For example, the caffeine week comes first because caffeine intake has been proven to put both dramatic short- and long-term stress on your body. Caffeine affects your metabolism in so many ways that it can make it almost impossible to deal effectively with sugar and nicotine and diet. But once you give it up, you can move on to these more difficult challenges with an altered metabolism that will help you succeed. Similarly, the sugar week comes before the smoking week. That's because a nicotine high may compensate for or be similar to a sugar high as far as your body is concerned, and if you try to give up smoking without modifying the amount of sugar in your diet, you'll find it very difficult to kick the habit. Likewise, you must improve your basic nutrition before you begin to take vitamin supplements. Vitamins and minerals are not, as too many people believe, substitutes for good nutrition; and if you take them for that reason, you'll be doing yourself more harm than good. Therefore, the nutrition-improvement week comes before the vitamin-mineral-supplement week.

Biochemical Boosters

Throughout the Medical Makeover, you'll be adding vitamins and minerals that will help you with each week's change. For example, you will take certain nutritional supplements that will enable you to handle stress better and therefore reduce your dependence on stimulants such as caffeine.

The biochemical boosters will help you where willpower has failed in the past. As your metabolism is altered, the changes you're making will be easy to stick with. The biochemical boosters are the key to breaking the addictions that are keeping you from enjoying optimum health.

Psychological and Physiological Approach

Most self-improvement programs depend on either a psychological or a physiological approach.

The most popular psychological approaches assume that the problem is with your mind. They depend on behavioral modification to get you to change your habits.

The physiological approaches hold that your body alone is the key. They emphasize a change of diet or adding vitamin and mineral supplements to make you feel better.

The Medical Makeover is the first program to combine both approaches. It doesn't depend entirely on will-power for success.

The psychological approach of the Makeover has been proven effective with hard-core addicts. Since bad habits truly are addictions, this approach will work for you. You'll learn some simple techniques that will help you change the behavior patterns that are taking a toll on your health. For example, you'll learn how to plan in advance, how to enlist helpers, how to recognize and avoid triggers to your bad habits, and how to make substitutions that will reinforce good habits in place of bad.

The physiological approach of the Makeover involves gradually altering your biochemistry through changing your diet, and through vitamin and mineral intakes, exercise, and stress control.

You'll find that by dealing with the mind and body at the same time, you'll be able to make changes that may have been too difficult in the past.

Flexible Future

The Medical Makeover is not geared to making fanatics. It's a program that takes real life into consideration, including the demands of your career, your family, your social commitments, and the strength of your willpower. Fatigue, boredom, depression, stress can all make it difficult to stick with your program. But having a relapse isn't as important as how you deal with the relapse. If you're so devastated by failure that you call your good intentions into question, this is making things harder for yourself. But if you allow for an occasional relapse and treat it as nothing more than a slight misstep that teaches you something, then you're on the right track.

I don't expect to make health fanatics—nor do I want to—of the people who go through the program. I realize the Makeover has to be compatible with the flow of one's life or it won't work for large numbers of people. I've tried to make it flexible enough so that the changes you're asked to make fit smoothly into your life-style.

How to Use the Medical Makeover

Here are some things you should know before you begin your Makeover:

1. The Medical Makeover is designed to be used over a period of eight weeks. Each week deals with a new health area.

2. Because the sequence of the weeks is so interdependent, it's important that you follow the order as given. Except for the weeks that you may skip, don't move ahead until you've completed each week in turn. And, by the way, if it takes you ten days or even two weeks to complete a step of the program, that's perfectly all right.

3. You don't need to read the entire book in advance. I do suggest that you read up to page 49 (which begins the first week) before you start so you understand some of the concepts of the Makeover. Otherwise I suggest that you read each week as you come to it.

4. Most of my patients find it easiest to begin a new Makeover week on a weekend. They find they have more time to prepare that way and are in the best psychological frame of mind. I suggest you do the same. Read about each new week on Thursday or Friday and do any preparation, including the questionnaires or any shopping, at that time (or on Saturday if that's the only time

you have). Then begin the week on either Saturday or Sunday. This will give you a bit of a head start on making the changes before you begin another week of routines, which can sometimes make change difficult.

Easing into the Makeover

Before you begin the first week of your Makeover, you are going to give your body a head start. You're going to begin to fight the pervasive effects of stress on your body. For most people, stress is a major factor keeping them from enjoying complete health. Not only that, stress could be what's preventing you from sticking to a diet or giving up smoking. After I explain how important to the Makeover fighting stress is, I'm going to recommend some vitamins that will get you in the best possible shape to begin the Makeover.

Stress: The Link Between Life-style and Disease

If you think of stress as something that happens mostly in your mind and that affects just your sense of calm and tranquillity, then you have an old-fashioned notion of stress—one that might be killing you. Important new research has demonstrated that stress is a component of all disease states, from the most mild fatigue to the most

34

serious chronic ailments, like cardiovascular disease. It affects not only your state of mind, but also your daily and long-term health.

It's important to understand the crucial connection between stress and most of your bad habits, including eating sweets, drinking coffee, drinking alcohol, and smoking. Stress could be the missing link in your previous efforts to lose weight, quit smoking, or cut down on your drinking.

The Risks of Stress Addiction

Many of my patients think that the ability to endure punishing amounts of job-related stress is an emblem of today's successful people—those who live life to the full and push to achieve their goals, whatever the personal cost. They are proud of having no spare time, of being astonishingly busy. The daily stress these people live with becomes almost an addiction. In fact, as we'll soon see, stress can be a physical addiction.

Like any addiction that keeps you from complete health, stress is one of the most significant links in the chain that leads to premature aging and general physical deterioration. For example, of all the risk factors in cardiovascular disease prevention, stress is one of the most pervasive. Stress can be associated with almost any other ailment, but the most common include cancer, diabetes, rheumatoid arthritis, peptic ulcers, and ulcerative colitis, bronchial asthma, headaches, and back pain. Of course, before these chronic diseases develop, your body goes through stages of deterioration during which you suffer from all the common minor symptoms that we've been discussing, including:

- tension headaches
- a constant sense of anxiety

- insomnia
- a feeling of constant tension
- complete exhaustion at the end of the day
- an inability to concentrate
- irritability
- frequent indigestion
- frequent constipation
- frequent colds

These are only the short-term effects of chronic unmanaged stress. The long-term effects include serious debilitating diseases. The actual effects of unmanaged stress on the body over a prolonged period include:

- chronic elevation of blood pressure with eventual damage to your heart, kidneys, and entire cardiovascular system.
- tearing of the arterial walls and elevation of the clotting elements in your blood, both of which increase plaque formation and thereby clog your arteries.
- changes in blood-sugar levels, and increases in your cholesterol levels.
- lowered resistance to disease because of a reduction in certain critically important white-blood-cell levels.
- increases in stomach acidity and changes in the stomach lining, which contribute to gastrointestinal distress and ulcer formation.
- inflammation in joints, aches and pains, and, ultimately, chronic arthritis.
- hyperactivity of the whole system, resulting in mental and physical exhaustion, chronic fatigue, and insomnia.

It's easy to see that chronic stress, when ignored, can contribute to sickness and death. When you become addicted to stress, and addicted also to stimulants that help you maintain the illusion of equilibrium, you are traveling in a truly vicious circle.

Toward the end of your Medical Makeover, we'll work on methods of stress management. Managing stress is a learned skill that will increase your sense of well-being dramatically as well as improve your overall health. For now, I want to make clear the connection, especially the **biochemical connection,** between stress and other bad habits.

Stress: Primitive Reaction to a Modern World

The body is constantly making an effort to maintain internal stability. This is called "homeostasis." The body will always do what it can to return to stability if that state is altered. Are you familiar with the big plastic clowns with sand in the base that children play with? No matter how hard or in what direction you push the clowns, they return to an upright position. So it is with the body; it's always working to return to a certain balanced state. If it's a very hot day, the body perspires to cool itself. If a bone is broken, the body works to mend it. The body creates scar tissue over a cut to protect itself from further damage, and it produces white blood cells to fight infections. Homeostatic activities include everything from the replacement of the lining of the digestive tract to the regulation of a woman's menstrual cycle. You depend on homeostatic activities for your health, and if one of your homeostatic systems breaks down, the result will be disease and perhaps death.

The body's response to stress is also an effort at homeostasis. Something—a stressor—acts upon your body, and you react with a complex series of biochemical changes that attempt to bring the body back into its prestressed state. It seems at first blush like a simple idea, but its ramifications in respect to maintaining health are awesome; indeed, many scientists consider stress theory to be one of the greatest contributions to the understanding of disease made in this century.

Dr. Hans Selye, the father of stress theory, defined stress as "the body's non-specific response to any demand made upon it." In simplest terms then, stress refers to everyday wear and tear on the body. Any physical or emotional demand from a broken leg to an invading virus to a sexual encounter involves stress. The stressor can be physical or emotional. Whether the stressor is a barking dog, a surprise party, a lost key, a reunion with an old friend, or even just the anticipation of a business meeting, your body prepares to meet the challenge in a variety of ways.

When the body is stressed, it reacts with a storm of biochemical responses, most significant being that the adrenal glands secrete various hormones, including the antistress hormones epinephrine and norepinephrine. These substances help the body mobilize energy to cope with the stress. This mobilization of energy is commonly known as the "fight or flight" response because the body is preparing to react in a decisive, physical fashion to the threat or stress.

Epinephrine and norepinephrine are responsible for a whole series of activities that occur immediately after the body is subject to stress. These antistress hormones heighten the nervous system's sensitivity, quicken the heartbeat, and sharpen the reflexes. The muscles tense, pupils dilate. The blood vessels of the skin contract so as to retain body heat and to force more blood into the major organs of the body. The liver releases stored glucose for energy to fight the stress. The digestive tract ceases its normal activity, also to conserve energy to fight the stress. The ability of the blood to coagulate is increased: In case the stress is a severe wound, the body will be able to prevent too great a loss of blood.

These responses would really be more appropriate for a caveman confronting a dinosaur than for a modern driver stuck in a traffic jam. For example, the fact that our pupils dilate as a result of stress is thought to have been crucial to primitive man's ability to see danger in a dark cave. It's hardly going to help us cope with the stress of urban noise. Likewise, we don't need our blood to coagulate more readily when we receive a promotion or news of a death in the family. But this biochemical response to stress is beyond our control. Part of our genetic code, it assumes that all stress will result in fear and flight; thus, it's a primitive reaction to a modern world.

Stress Exhaustion

Most stressors we experience don't demand a physical reaction. What does the body do about all the changes that are not necessary to escape the stress?

If the stressor is a specific, limited event like a skid on an icy road, the body recovers once the event is over. It replenishes its energy stores and returns to its optimum state of homeostasis. Recharged and replenished, the body will be ready to meet the next stress imposed upon it. Unfortunately, this is a sort of "ideal" stress; it's more common to be assaulted by a constant, unremitting battery of stressors that don't have clear beginnings, middles, and ends.

If the stress is the constant anxiety over job performance or the trauma of an unhappy marriage, then the body has no opportunity to restore its reserves. It goes into what Selye called the "stage of resistance," or adaptation, where it tries to adjust to the constant stress. The stage of resistance is useful for coping with long-term stress like a severe illness or injury or severe hardships. But for the kind of constant stress most of us endure daily, it's overkill. Eventually, in the face of unremitting stress, the body will enter the "exhaustion stage." It is so exhausted from the continual resistance to the stress that it can no longer function properly. At this stage you begin to exhibit the vague symptoms I discussed previously—the headaches, lethargy, inability to concentrate, etc., that are keeping you from enjoying complete health.

Why Your Body Needs Help to Fight Stress

The body fights stress with two types of energy, which Selye named "superficial" and "adaptation" energy.

The superficial energy can be replaced. Good nutrition, exercise, the right vitamins and minerals, relaxation techniques, and eliminating caffeine, alcohol, and smoking will all help reduce the drain of your superficial energy.

Eventually, however, you're fighting a losing battle if you don't deal with the source of stress itself. You can replenish your body only to a certain degree; then the superficial energy runs out and you begin to draw on the adaptation energy. At this point, you're dealing with a limited resource, and Selye and others believe that when this finite reserve of adaptation energy is used up that senility and death result.

It's a generally accepted part of the medical canon that people in high-stress jobs will be more disease prone, and will age more quickly than people under less stress. Perhaps you've seen photographs of national politicians taken before and after a four-year term in office. In many cases, the aging that shows in the faces of people under such constant stress is dramatic. They are people who are spending a great deal of their irreplaceable adaptation energy in a single spurt.

The amount of adaptation energy that you yourself have cannot be determined. Experiments with animals have demonstrated that reserves of adaptation energy are finite and are genetically determined. A research study showed that if you expose rats to cold water, they can tolerate it for a certain amount of time. If you repeatedly expose them to cold water, the rats will eventually be able to tolerate it for longer and longer periods. But finally they will reach a point, which differs slightly with each rat, depending on its genetic heritage, where it can no longer cope with the cold water. Physical deterioration and death will then result.

The same is true for people: We all have a certain amount of adaptation energy; how much is the question. Keeping it in reserve and relying on superficial energy to deal with stress will keep you healthy a lot longer than constantly drawing on your adaptation energy. The more you can conserve your adaptation energy, the better. This is the central concept of the Medical Makeover program. It is designed to replenish and conserve your superficial energy so that your adaptation energy will last as long as possible.

Stress and Your Bad Habits

The antistress hormones epinephrine and norepinephrine, which are released by the body in response to stress, are powerful substances. Epinephrine acts quickly to prepare the body for the fight-or-flight response and all its physiological changes that the response entails— from dilation of the pupils to tensing of the muscles to constriction of the blood vessels. An important result of the release of epinephrine is that as it travels through the liver, it causes glucose to be released into the blood. This glucose provides the energy the body uses to fight or flee. But for modern man, who is probably not fighting or fleeing but rather boiling quietly in a state of rage or concern, the release of glucose creates a complex problem.

In many people over a period of time, the body's

ability to release glucose into the bloodstream becomes impaired because of exhaustion of the body's natural ability. When this happens, the glucose level in the blood does not rise and the body continues to release norepinephrine and epinephrine in an effort to supply the missing glucose. You feel this increased release of epinephrine and norepinephrine as anxiety or nervousness. At the same time, the hormone is still decreasing the blood flow to your skin, making you feel cool and causing your mouth to feel dry, among other things. These physical changes can stimulate you to want to have a drink, something to eat, or a cigarette. For example, stress can cause the body to release appetite-stimulating substances that will cause you to overeat. The nervousness that results when norepinephrine is released can make some people overeat and others drink compulsively. Stress can cause smokers to smoke even more heavily. Stress therefore is actually encouraging the development of bad habits.

The release of the antistress hormones is intended to give you a boost of energy, and it does. But when that boost wears off, you feel more tired than ever.

Perhaps you've experienced having to speak in public. Most people feel very anxious beforehand; so as your body faces this stress, it's producing norepinephrine, which, among other things, is tensing the muscles, drying the mouth, perhaps causing diarrhea, and giving you an extra boost of energy.

But remember how you feel when the speech is over at last? Relieved and exhilarated, yes; but also, after a short time, exhausted. The stressor—the speech—has drained your body of energy reserves and you're feeling let down. It's at this point that you crave a stimulant—something to bring you up to that high-energy state you were in as a result of stress. Perhaps you'll have a cup of coffee or even a cigarette. All these things elevate the secretion of norepinephrine in your body and simulate the boost you felt when you were stressed.

Over a period of time you learn, on a subconscious level at least, that you feel best when you're stimulated and because so much of the time the stimulation is caused by the stress in your life, you fight to maintain that energy level artificially. Over a period of time many of my patients have so depleted their energy reserves through a combination of stress and bad habits that they no longer know what it feels like to enjoy a natural bountiful reserve of energy with which to meet the challenges of daily life. They're completely addicted to artificial stimulants and don't even know it. Over the years they've become physiologically programmed to develop bad habits, and once programmed, they have found it almost impossible to change.

It seems that many people (certainly many of my patients) develop a taste for coffee, cigarettes, and sweets at a stage in their lives when they begin to feel regular stress. Perhaps they began to drink coffee and to smoke cigarettes in school. The food was terrible and their class schedule was demanding, so they relied on candy bars as quick snacks. When they prepared for an exam or finished a paper, they smoked and drank even more coffee than usual. By the time they became engrossed in careers that demanded that they adapt to new, ever higher levels of stress, they were quite dependent on coffee and sugar and cigarettes to keep them "up."

But, the body can't continue to release unlimited quantities of epinephrine, norepinephrine, glucose, and other substances that stress depletes. Indeed, the body can only store a day's worth of glucose to be derived from the liver, and once that amount is used up, the body will draw upon the muscles for additional supplies. Eventually the body becomes exhausted by the biochemical demands of stress. When you reach this stage, you're burning the candle at both ends. The body's waning ability to cope with stress biochemically as its reserves become depleted reinforces the bad habits that, in the short term, help you "feel normal." By now you're running fast on a treadmill, getting nowhere. As your body becomes more and more exhausted, you become more and more dependent on stimulants to keep it going.

So many patients have told me that no matter what they've tried, they can't stick to a diet or cut down on their drinking or give up smoking. When they've tried, when they've told themselves that it's time to shape up, their usual course of action has been to abruptly give up all their bad habits. But when they do, because they've been overstimulated for so long, they feel absolutely awful. Suddenly what they have done to themselves for months or years is revealed and previously disguised problems are unmasked. Most people simply can't take the discomfort of these feelings, and so either they drop their self-improvement plans at the first temptation or they gradually work their way back by having "just a little pick-me-up" in the morning and a tiny drink at night until they're right back where they started.

The Secret Stress

There's another secret stress that affects your health. As we've seen, a stress can come from an external physical threat or from an emotional reaction to an imagined threat. But stress can be caused by the body's reaction to stress itself! Like the question of which came first, the chicken or the egg, there's little point in separating these two responses; it's enough to know how they affect your body.

When your body mobilizes to fight a stress, the liver converts stored sugar into glucose so a ready source of energy is available. If this glucose is not in an amount that the body deems sufficient to cope with the stress—most likely because of depleted reserves—then the body perceives this lack of glucose as a stress in and of itself. Thus, the stress response is intensified and the body's reserves further depleted.

You may be aware of many of the ways in which your body responds to stress. You feel your hands getting clammy, you feel an increase in perspiration, you're well aware of a sense of anxiety and nervousness. But the biochemical stress that is a result of stress itself is hidden. If you're run down to begin with, this hidden stress has been doing its damage over the years and is multiplying the bad effects of stress you're already suffering.

Prepping for the Makeover

Consultation after consultation with thousands of patients have led me to the following conclusion: There is a biochemical state that corresponds with feeling "run down," and this state is in fact an exhaustion of the body's ability to manufacture antistress hormones and a corresponding loss of its ability to cope with the damaging effects of stress. The goal of the Medical Makeover is to augment your ability to synthesize these antistress hormones and to prevent the biochemical disturbances caused by stress. Once you've achieved this, you'll find it much easier to break your bad habits. Certain vitamin and mineral supplements augment your ability to produce these antistress hormones and help you resist the damaging effects of stress.

One of the ways that stress debilitates you is by lessening your ability to deactivate certain damaging molecules called "free radicals." It is thought that free-radical reactions underlie many of the biochemical disturbances that result in cell injury, inflammation, and consequent degenerative disease states, including cancer. Convincing studies done with both animals and humans show that this free-radical damage can be prevented by taking certain vitamins and minerals called "antioxidants." They enable us to adapt to stress better and help us live longer, healthier lives.

I've found that my patients who take antioxidants are better able to cope with stress and have fewer vague symptoms. At the same time, the antioxidants help them resist addictions to caffeine, alcohol, etc. You should begin taking these vitamins and minerals immediately, even if you don't begin the Makeover for another few days. Here is the antistress formula that I recommend:

A good-quality multiple vitamin and mineral compound containing 10,000 IUs of beta-carotene and approximately 50 mg. of each of the B vitamins plus Vitamin C: 1,000 mg.
Vitamin E: 400 IUs
Selenium: 50 mcg.

You see now how stress can start a chain reaction that results in the development of bad habits and the degeneration of health. Stress comes into play during each week of the Medical Makeover. It's the linchpin that links behavior and disease. In the stress-management week, we'll work on techniques that have proven effective in fighting stress, because only by managing stress can you become truly healthy.

PART II

THE PROGRAM

Week One: Caffeine

One of the first and biggest obstacles to overcoming an addiction is acknowledging you have one. I've found that for most of my patients, recognizing the reality and significance of their caffeine addiction is more difficult than actually giving it up. In fact, when a regular coffee drinker agrees, with no comment or protest whatsoever, to give up coffee completely, I'm always a little suspicious. And I make a point to explain in some detail why caffeine must be completely eliminated from the diet. Otherwise, I know that these people are telling themselves that having one or two cups of coffee or tea surely won't make any difference.

Barbara M. was one of these secretly reluctant patients. When I announced that giving up caffeine was crucial to the success of the Medical Makeover, she silently drew a line in her mind: Everything else she would do, but giving up coffee was asking too much. Barbara had begun her coffee habit several years ago by drinking one or two cups a day. Then she worked up to about ten cups a day and couldn't imagine life without coffee. It got her going in the morning and kept her going through the day. Though she wouldn't admit it until later, she subconsciously ascribed some of her success—she is a features editor for a well-known national women's fashion magazine—to the energy that coffee gave her. By the time Barbara came to see me it was obvious she was using caffeine as a stimulant because she felt so sick. She had frequent headaches and, between cups of coffee, was absolutely exhausted.

Barbara first tried cutting down to three cups a day. She still felt terrible because the coffee was causing her to crave the cups she had cut out. She would get a rush from the first cup in the morning, and when that wore off, she would want more caffeine to get that temporary high. Eventually, as I talked to her week after week about how caffeine was altering her metabolism, she stopped completely. She had intense withdrawal symptoms the first week. She would have a headache in the late morning and another in the afternoon. Her muscles ached and she had severe neck and shoulder pains. Only after she experienced caffeine withdrawal was she able to realize the severity of her addiction and begin to appreciate the effect it was having on her overall health.

This Week's Goal

The first goal in your Medical Makeover will be to eliminate caffeine from your diet. You should be able to do this easily within a week. By cutting out caffeine you will be making the first move to stop the process of deterioration that you may experience as headaches, afternoon fatigue, anxiety, nervousness, and insomnia. You will halt the loss of vitamins and minerals that caffeine causes, and you will help avoid the chronic, long-term diseases that have been linked to caffeine. You should feel the results, which my patients usually report as a new feeling of calm and increased energy, by the end of the first week.

The first part of this chapter will explain to you the effects of caffeine on your body. If you don't know the facts, you'll be tempted either to skip this week or to backslide once the good effects of the Makeover begin to be felt. When you learn how bad caffeine is for you, coupled with the withdrawal you'll probably experience, you'll appreciate the intimate connection between your health and your habits. Like my patients, you'll feel a sense of mastery that will carry you through into the next challenge of the Medical Makeover.

Although there are compelling biochemical reasons for eliminating caffeine as the first step of the Medical Makeover, I've discovered in my practice that paying attention to the effects of caffeine on the body, despite the popularity of caffeine today, is a powerful incentive for my patients. It's a relatively easy addiction to break, despite what you might think. It's also an important beginning to developing a new consciousness of health as a personal, individual, achievable goal.

Before you decide you can skip this first week of the Makeover because you don't drink coffee or tea, be sure to check the table on pages 64–66 for the caffeine content of major foods and over-the-counter drugs. Many everyday medications contain large amounts of caffeine, which can trap you into becoming an addict. One of the worst cases of caffeine addiction I ever encountered was a man who drank very little coffee but took daily doses of Excedrin which gave him a "hidden" caffeine intake in amounts exceeding that contained in eight cups of coffee.

The second part of this chapter will tell you exactly how to go about giving up caffeine. This doesn't mean you'll never again be able to have a cup of coffee—that day *will* come—but first you'll have to break your addiction to it.

Caffeine: The Respectable Addiction

It's easy to see why people are so reluctant to give up caffeine: It's a socially sanctioned addiction, and most of us are unaware that it's an addiction in the first place. Coffee advertising encourages people to view having a cup of coffee as a boost in the morning, a pick-me-up at midday, a gratifying way to end a fine dinner, and most bizarrely, given the powerful effects of caffeine on the nervous system, an opportunity for a relaxing interlude in an otherwise frantic day. In an effort to lure young coffee drinkers, advertising has touted coffee as the "drink of success," implying that you work hard, exercise, eat light, and keep it all perking along with coffee. The truth is something else again.

The Department of Health, Education and Welfare lists caffeine as addictive, along with nicotine and heroin, and admits that if caffeine were a new drug, the manufacturer would have great difficulty in getting a license to sell it, and it would no doubt be available only by prescription.

Coffee drinkers experience the three distinct signs of addiction: tolerance for the drug, withdrawal symptoms when it is removed, and a craving after being deprived. The director of the FDA's Bureau of Foods has stated, "We're not saying it's unsafe; we're just not saying it's safe."

But it is unsafe. The data increasingly show that caffeine is implicated in several types of cancer, including leukemia and pancreatic cancer, one of the most common and most often fatal types. For men, it may be related to cancer of the prostate and intestines; for women, to lung, larynx, breast, and ovarian cancer. Even drinking one or two cups a day increases the risk.

While most cystic breast tumors are not cancerous, women who have them may be more likely to develop breast cancer eventually; and coffee is clearly implicated in breast cysts. An Ohio State University study of women who completely eliminated caffeine from their diet found that within six months, 65 percent of them no longer had breast cysts. I've had similar success with women whose breast cysts disappeared once they eliminated all caffeine from their diet.

The data on heart disease and coffee are just as damning; this is not surprising since we all experience some difference in heart rhythm after as little as two cups of coffee. Over a period of time, regular coffee drinkers are frequently subject to various cardiac irregularities. One study found a link between coffee and heart attacks. That may be partly because coffee drinkers are more likely to have high blood levels of cholesterol, which also increases the probability of heart disease.

Additionally, caffeine is implicated in high blood pressure—if you're a borderline case, caffeine may tip the scale—and many other disorders, including peptic ulcer, diabetes, psychosis, and birth defects.

Caffeinism

It is the immediate effects of caffeine that concern us the most in the Makeover. Recent studies have linked *caffeinism* to anxiety, restlessness, agitation, muscle tremors, headaches, sensory disturbances, cardiovascular symptoms, and gastrointestinal complaints. Caffeinism can result from an intake of 500 to 600 milligrams of caffeine per day, which is approximately two to four cups of coffee, or seven to nine cups of tea. I've seen similar symptoms in patients who drink two or three cups of coffee per day.

Although infrequently diagnosed, caffeinism is described as a significant health risk. It is frequently the real problem when a patient is diagnosed as having an "anxiety neurosis"; and the recognition of this growing problem led to caffeinism being included in the *Diagnostic and Statistical Manual (III)* of the American Psychiatric Association.

Despite these sobering facts, an estimated ninety million Americans consume six or seven cups a day—enough to make caffeinism a national disease. Many soft drinks—which are consumed in such vast quantities that they provide up to one tenth of the total calories in some diets—provide caffeine that is nearly the equal of an average adult's coffee consumption. The average American, including children, consumes roughly 200 milligrams of caffeine each day—double the amount it takes to affect the body significantly. Twenty to 30 percent of us consume more than 500 milligrams of caffeine daily, which is double what doctors consider a large "drug dose." Ten percent of us ingest more than 1,000 milligrams each day.

I don't mean to exaggerate or sensationalize the dangers of caffeine ingestion. But we can't ignore its short- and long-term effects, which most of us are unaware of and that affect our everyday health and well-being as well as our future health.

Caffeine: The Quicker Picker-Upper

Caffeine is a stimulant that's been around for thousands of years. Though it has been "domesticated," in that it has become part of our everyday lives, when the stimulating qualities of coffee were first discovered, its use was restricted to religious ceremonies. In the Middle East it enabled Muslims to stay up all night praying and chanting. Caffeine—in the form of coffee—eventually became popular all over the world for the same reason it is held in high esteem today: its stimulating action.

Caffeine is a member of the drug family known as stimulants. All stimulants act on the body in a similar way. They encourage the body to release epinephrine and norepinephrine, the antistress hormones mentioned previously in relation to stress. With the release of the antistress hormones, the body feels the familiar sensations. The heart beats faster, the blood pressure rises, the stomach jumps, the bowels may react, and the blood vessels constrict.

While you may not be aware of what is happening internally, you are probably familiar with these sensations: a sense of energy, increased urine output, bowel movements, and cold extremities. These effects may be felt within minutes after taking caffeine and reach their peak in an hour to an hour and a half, finally tapering off after about three and a half hours. Some people feel the effects of caffeine for a much longer time.

Although most of my patients are willing to admit that caffeine is a stimulant, they're less likely to recognize that it is responsible for a host of other irritations that they ascribe to "nerves," or "stress," or just "a hard day at the office." These complaints include insomnia, headaches, irritability, heart palpitations, feelings of disorientation, and nausea. Stomach irritation, heartburn, and indigestion are also commonly caused by caffeine.

Among different individuals, the metabolic half-life of caffeine, or the length of time that its effects are felt in the system, varies considerably—by as much as four to ten hours. This means that, depending on your metabolism, your morning cup of coffee could wear off at 10:00 A.M., noon, or dinnertime, and the coffee or cola you drink in the afternoon could still be affecting your body at 3:00 A.M. Because of this variation in the way people react to caffeine, some never connect the symptoms of caffeine withdrawal to coffee, tea, or cola consumption. If you have just one cup of coffee in the morning, it may never occur to you that your early-afternoon headache is the result of the caffeine wearing off. If then you take a pain reliever containing caffeine, your headache may go away with the introduction of the drug into your system, but in the morning you'll crave that cup of coffee as you begin to feel withdrawal symptoms again.

A common syndrome among my coffee-drinking patients is to have three, four, or five cups during the day and perhaps a cola drink or two. They claim to feel no adverse effects from all this caffeine, but they wake up every morning with a slight, and in some cases severe, headache. It's only when they give up caffeine completely that they really believe my diagnosis: daily withdrawal. Every morning, after hours of sleep with no caffeine, their bodies undergo withdrawal with the most common symptom—a headache. Once they have their morning cup of coffee—their fix—the headache goes away, and they begin the cycle all over again. As with other addictions, once your body grows accustomed to caffeine, you must take regular, fairly precise doses to stay on an even keel. Too much or too little will result in uncomfortable symptoms.

The individual variations in the way caffeine is metabolized by your body, coupled with the different levels of addiction, could account for the differing effects it has on sleep patterns. There's no doubt that caffeine affects your sleep, whether you know it or not. Heavy coffee drinkers may not experience the trouble falling asleep that light coffee drinkers suffer from, though the same heavy coffee drinkers may sleep less soundly.

Because caffeine is metabolized differently by different people, caffeine addicts can experience problems with prescription drugs. Birth control pills cause high retention and slower elimination of caffeine. Equanil and Miltown may delay elimination of caffeine from the body and cause concentration of caffeine in the brain. Asthma medications may cause excessive nervousness if taken with caffeine. And nicotine doubles the rate at which the body metabolizes caffeine, which may double the amount of caffeine desired by smokers. And there may be many other drug-caffeine interactions that we don't know about.

Caffeine and Energy

Caffeine rushes through the body, affecting the brain, the central nervous system, the heart and circulatory system, the respiratory system, and the digestive tract. Caffeine has been linked with diseases and disorders in all these systems, but for my patients, its effects on energy and stress are the most immediately troublesome.

The main appeal of caffeine is its ability to give an energy boost. But that energy boost is actually deceptive. Caffeine doesn't give you extra energy; it just forces the body to deplete its reserve of energy faster than it would otherwise. When caffeine is absorbed into the system, the body is stimulated, the mind feels more alert, fatigue is vanquished. A mug of coffee contains enough caffeine to raise the metabolism 10 to 25 percent, which is the equivalent of 10 milligrams of amphetamine. The body goes into overdrive. But when the effects of the caffeine wear off, in two and a half to three or four hours, the body feels the effects of having drawn on its energy reserves. It goes into a slump and feels more fatigued than ever.

In my experience, patients who are caffeine addicts rarely notice this slump because their constant consumption manages to keep them revved up. It's when they give up caffeine that they notice the high-low cycle. Barbara M., the magazine editor we met at the beginning of this chapter, said that a few weeks after she had given up caffeine she went to an early-morning editorial seminar at a midtown hotel. The coffee being passed around smelled so good that she just couldn't resist one cup. She was so engrossed in the seminar that at first she was oblivious to the effects of the caffeine. But within an hour after drinking the coffee, she said she felt uncomfortably hyper and irritable.

Barbara's body had adjusted to a normal metabolism without caffeine, so now its effects were much more powerful. This didn't surprise her, but she didn't like the feeling and wasn't eager to repeat it. What did surprise her was that by lunchtime she was exhausted. She could barely concentrate on the last discussion group and could think of nothing except how much she wanted a nap. When the group broke for lunch, Barbara found an empty meeting room and stretched out for a catnap, only to find that though her body was exhausted, her mind was still racing from the caffeine. She said the whole experience was a shock, and if she hadn't been aware of how caffeine affects the body and hadn't given it up for those few weeks, she would never have appreciated that a single cup of coffee had ruined her morning.

The low that follows caffeine ingestion is the very reason the substance is so addictive. When you feel that familiar slump, your instinct is to get another jump start from another cup of coffee. So the cycle continues until your normal metabolism and normal biochemistry are completely awry.

Caffeine and Performance

If people did not become addicted to caffeine and therefore not driven by a powerful physiological need, would they continue to drink coffee? Though we can't really separate cause and effect in the cycle of caffeine addiction, I believe that most people would still be attracted to caffeine. Aside from the energy boost it provides, the majority believe that it improves their performance, which is the one undesirable advantage of caffeine cited in most every discussion of its effects. A study that supports this idea found that typists improved speed and efficiency after ingesting caffeine. But further studies reveal that faster typing doesn't tell the whole story.

The stimulating effects of caffeine would surely point to better performance, but when you take into account the increasing arousal and anxiety it also produces, you've moved one step forward and two steps back. A summary of caffeine and performance studies found that caffeine does improve mental acuity in simple arithmetic and typing, and in uncoding. It also increases your ability to do exhausting work, whether long-distance driving or assembly-line manufacturing. But caffeine can result in hand tremors and possible difficulties with eye-hand coordination. Worst of all, from the point of view of most people who depend on caffeine to improve their work performance, studies have shown that it can have an unpredictable effect on tasks involving choice and discrimination. In one study of college students it was discovered that those with a high consumption of caffeine had lower achievement and grades than those with a low caffeine intake. The implication is that if you are doing work that demands choice and discrimination, caffeine may not be giving you as much help as you think.

Caffeine: The Diet Killer

The fatigue you experience as your body realigns its metabolism following caffeine ingestion may be largely the result of low blood sugar. We'll examine this problem in detail during the sugar week. For now it's important for you to know that low blood sugar masked by caffeine ingestion, in addition to taxing the body's energy reserves, can be a trap for dieters.

Many dieters depend on caffeine to depress their appetites, and it's true that this is one of its effects. But in the long run, drinking a lot of coffee makes dieters more vulnerable to attacks of hunger resulting from low blood sugar.

One of the effects of caffeine is to release hormones that force the body to release stored glycogen from the liver in the form of glucose. You experience this as a boost in energy as the glucose flows into the bloodstream and the body is stimulated to release insulin. The flood of insulin depresses the level of glucose, but as this level plummets, the body reacts with a low, or a slump. The increased blood sugar that was giving you that rush of energy is depressed now to even lower levels and you feel tired, irritable, and, most troublesome for dieters, famished.

From a practical standpoint, it's these hunger attacks that always seem to drive dieters to break down and have a chocolate éclair, which does enormous harm from a physiological as well as a psychological standpoint. The body cries out for a snack to get that blood sugar up again, and most people receive this message as a desperate plea for something sweet. If you indulge, the cycle continues. Therefore, coffee, instead of being a crutch for dieters, is in fact a trap. If you want to raise your metabolism to lose weight, you would do better to eat a good breakfast. Studies have shown that a good balanced breakfast increases your metabolism by about 14 percent!

Dieters can exacerbate their caffeine addiction as well as their diet plans with over-the-counter diet pills. Many of these diet pills typically contain up to 200 milligrams of caffeine—more than twice that found in an average cup of coffee. Certainly they will depress your appetite temporarily, but then the syndrome that I described above will occur. When the effects wear off, you will experience a raging hunger, to say nothing of the probable headache, nervousness, stomach irritation, and overall fatigue that are by-products of caffeine abuse. Taking these pills is a dangerous and usually fruitless approach to weight loss.

Caffeine and Stress

I know some of you still aren't convinced that you can give up coffee. How can you get through your stressful days, you ask. Let me emphasize that by taking caffeine you are only adding to your problem and contributing to a feeling of being generally run down. This is the way it works.

Every time we drink a cup of coffee, or have a soda with caffeine in it, or a cup of tea, we are stimulating our adrenal glands to release the antistress hormones. Coffee also causes an immediate, temporary, rise in blood sugar. Both these biochemical reactions make us feel better temporarily. We find it's easier to deal with the kids, or the boss, or a busy schedule, or a work deadline, or any of the 101 minor irritations and strains that are part and parcel of our daily lives. And the more stress in our lives we perceive, the more likely we'll reach for a cup of coffee.

But metabolically there's no free lunch. In actuality, what we are forcing the body to do is deplete its reserves of antistress hormones. Because we've been using external stimulants to switch on our adrenal glands, and have not been relying on internal triggers, the adrenals become exhausted. We start feeling run down, worn out, exhausted, overwhelmed, and unable to cope. And what makes it seem like we can cope? As the TV commercials will be glad to tell you, it's another cup of coffee.

This is a major reason why it is so difficult to give up caffeine, and why we, as a nation, are so strongly addicted to it. When we don't have caffeine, our bodies don't produce naturally the catecholamines that make it easier to get through the day, to cope with city traffic, difficult children, job pressures. We have lost the ability to respond internally to stress without a stimulant.

Once we deny ourselves the caffeine, not only do we feel terrible, we begin experiencing withdrawal; this makes us feel even worse. That's why our will to give up caffeine so often fails when we try to get through a day, or a week, without it.

This is where nutritional supplements are helpful, particularly those vitamins and minerals known as antioxidants. They seem to increase naturally your ability to cope with stress, and therefore make it easier to give up your addictions. If you haven't started taking these supplements (as I suggested at the end of the chapter about stress), do so when you give up coffee. My antistress formula is given on page 46.

Caffeine: Habit or Addiction?

What role does caffeine play in your life? Here are some questions that will help you recognize whether caffeine is a habit, a dependence, or an addiction for you.

1. Do you need a cup of coffee to start the day?
2. Do you usually have a second cup before lunch?
3. Does it bother you if you miss your midmorning or midafternoon coffee break?
4. Do you drink more coffee when under stress?
5. Do you consume more than 250 milligrams of caffeine every day?
6. If you've ever gone a whole day without coffee or other caffeinated drink:

 —did you feel dramatically different?
 —did you drink more coffee the next day?
 —did you have a headache?

7. Do you always choose a coffee, tea, or cola that has caffeine rather than one that doesn't?
8. Do you regularly experience more than two of the recognized symptoms of caffeinism (insomnia, depres-

sion, irritability, chronic fatigue, restlessness, rapid pulse or heartbeat, stomach pains or heartburn, headaches, diarrhea, anxiety)?

9. Do you depend on coffee to make you feel good?
10. Do you think it's impossible to face the day without coffee?

If you answered yes to only the first two questions, you have a caffeine habit. If you answered yes to questions 1 through 4, you suffer from a caffeine dependence. If you answered yes to eight or more questions, you are addicted to caffeine.

Kicking Caffeine

Now it's time to plan your caffeine-free life. But, again, for those of you who are dismayed at the prospect of living the rest of your lives without another cup of coffee, it's not essential to give up caffeine forever. Unlike smoking, caffeine does not seem to be an all-or-nothing addiction. The day will come when you can have a cup of coffee or tea or a caffeinated cola with no dramatic ill effects. But first you must conquer the everyday, habitual addiction. I recommend that you completely eliminate caffeine from your diet for at least six weeks. Within one week you will begin to feel better, and within six weeks you should find any lingering desire for caffeine is gone. But don't begin this first step of the Medical Makeover with the idea that this is only a temporary change of pace; think of it as a total life change. In six weeks you'll be a different person, at least metabolically, and you may find that you'll never again feel the desire for caffeine in any form.

Taking Stock

Before you begin the caffeine week, you must know how much caffeine is contained in your diet. Even if you don't drink coffee or tea or carbonated beverages, you still need to check all the medications you take to learn if hidden caffeine has given you an addiction. One of my patients, suffering caffeine-withdrawal headaches, began to take a pain reliever. At first he took a few pills a day, but as his headaches became more regular, he was up to the maximum dosage. It wasn't until he discovered the pain reliever contained caffeine that he realized he hadn't kicked his caffeine addiction at all. He had exchanged pain relievers for coffee to get his daily fix.

The following table will help you figure out how much caffeine you're consuming. Be sure to check each item on the table that you might have on an ordinary day.

CAFFEINE COUNTDOWN:
Identifying the Sources of Caffeine in Your Diet*

Product	Amount	Milligrams	Total
Coffee (5-oz. cup)			
Brewed, drip method	_____ ×	115	= _____
Brewed, percolator	_____ ×	80	= _____
Instant	_____ ×	65	= _____
Decaffeinated, brewed	_____ ×	3	= _____
Decaffeinated, instant	_____ ×	2	= _____
Tea (5-oz. cup)			
Brewed, major U.S. brands	_____ ×	40	= _____
Brewed, imported brands	_____ ×	60	= _____
Instant	_____ ×	30	= _____
Iced (12-oz. glass)	_____ ×	70	= _____
Cocoa beverage (5-oz. cup)	_____ ×	4	= _____
Chocolate milk beverage (8 oz.)	_____ ×	5	= _____
Milk chocolate (1 oz.)	_____ ×	6	= _____

CAFFEINE COUNTDOWN:
Identifying the Sources of Caffeine in Your Diet*

Product	Amount		Milligrams		Total
Dark chocolate, semisweet					
(1 oz.)	_____	×	20	=	_____
Baker's chocolate (1 oz.)	_____	×	26	=	_____
Chocolate-flavored syrup					
(1 oz.)	_____	×	4	=	_____
Soft Drinks (12-oz. serving)					
Sugar-Free Mr. PIBB	_____	×	58.8	=	_____
Mountain Dew	_____	×	54.0	=	_____
Mello Yello	_____	×	52.8	=	_____
TAB	_____	×	46.8	=	_____
Coca-Cola	_____	×	45.6	=	_____
Diet Coke	_____	×	45.6	=	_____
Shasta Cola	_____	×	44.4	=	_____
Shasta Cherry Cola	_____	×	44.4	=	_____
Shasta Diet Cola	_____	×	44.4	=	_____
Mr. PIBB	_____	×	40.8	=	_____
Dr. Pepper	_____	×	39.6	=	_____
Sugar-Free Dr. Pepper	_____	×	39.6	=	_____
Big Red	_____	×	38.4	=	_____
Sugar-Free Big Red	_____	×	38.4	=	_____
Pepsi-Cola	_____	×	38.4	=	_____
Aspen	_____	×	36.0	=	_____
Diet Pepsi	_____	×	36.0	=	_____
Pepsi Light	_____	×	36.0	=	_____
RC Cola	_____	×	36.0	=	_____
Diet Rite	_____	×	36.0	=	_____
Kick	_____	×	31.2	=	_____
Canada Dry Jamaica Cola	_____	×	30.0	=	_____
Canada Dry Diet Cola	_____	×	1.2	=	_____
Drugs					
Prescription Drugs					
Cafergot (migraine)	_____	×	100	=	_____
Fiorinal (tension headache)	_____	×	40	=	_____
Darvon Compound (pain					
relief)	_____	×	32.4	=	_____

CAFFEINE COUNTDOWN:
Identifying the Sources of Caffeine in Your Diet*

Product	Amount	Milligrams	Total
Nonprescription Drugs			
Weight-control aids			
Codexin	_____	× 200	= _____
Dex-A-Diet II	_____	× 200	= _____
Dexatrim, Dexatrim Extra Strength	_____	× 200	= _____
Dietac Capsules	_____	× 200	= _____
Maximum Strength Appedrine	_____	× 100	= _____
Prolamine	_____	× 140	= _____
Alertness Tablets			
Nodoz	_____	× 100	= _____
Vivarin	_____	× 200	= _____
Analgesics/Pain Relievers			
Anacin, Maximum Strength Anacin	_____	× 32	= _____
Excedrin	_____	× 65	= _____
Midol	_____	× 32.4	= _____
Vanquish	_____	× 33	= _____
Diuretics			
Aqua-Ban	_____	× 100	= _____
Maximum Strength Aqua-Ban Plus	_____	× 200	= _____
Permathene H2 Off	_____	× 200	= _____
Cold and Allergy Remedies			
Coryban-D capsules	_____	× 30	= _____
Triaminicin tablets	_____	× 30	= _____
Dristan Decongestant tablets & Dristan A-F Decongestant tablets	_____	× 16.2	= _____
Duradyne-Forte tablets	_____	× 30	= _____
	Total Daily Caffeine		= _____

*Source: National Center for Drugs and Biologics, Food and Drug Administration, March 1984

Now that you know your total daily caffeine intake, you can assess what effect it's having on your body.

If you consume less than 300 milligrams daily, you may not be addicted to caffeine, but you may be suffering its effects. It probably has a subtle influence on your sleep patterns and your energy levels throughout the day.

If you consume 300 milligrams or more daily, you may have psychological and physiological dependencies on caffeine. You are also at twice the risk for developing ulcers, and, if you are a woman, fibrocystic disease. You are also robbing your body of essential vitamins and minerals, particularly if you are a woman.

If you consume 600 milligrams or more daily, you may be addicted to caffeine. You double your risk of heart attack, and you probably suffer from at least some, if not all, of the symptoms of caffeinism (see page 62).

If you consume 1,000 milligrams or more daily, you are addicted to caffeine, probably suffer from many of the symptoms of caffeinism (see page 62), and you are in danger of developing heart disease, cancer, ulcers, or even mental illness.

Cold Turkey or the Step-by-Step Approach?

Many of my patients ask if they can just taper off their caffeine consumption before quitting completely. Though some experts recommend a gradual tapering-off, I've found the cold-turkey method to be far preferable. Most of my patients who tried the gradual approach found it more difficult because it was harder to know when to draw the line. Were two cups a day acceptable if they cut down from six? Or should they try for one? As long as they had just two cups, did it really matter if they had one more after dinner as long as they were lingering with friends in a nice restaurant? When the process of quitting becomes one of constant decision-making, resolve is inevitably weakened.

There's also a physiological reason for quitting cold turkey. It's just too difficult to see the effects of eliminating caffeine from your diet if you are still consuming even a small amount. You'll still have those energy swings and perhaps many of your vague symptoms under these conditions, and you'll have less incentive to stick with your resolution to quit completely. Moreover, the lingering physical effects of caffeine will weaken your determination. Caffeine has been shown to cause depression and fatigue. This makes any self-improvement program more difficult to stick with, and, especially at the beginning of the Medical Makeover, I think you should make things as easy for yourself as you can.

What About Decaf?

I ask all my patients to abstain from decaffeinated teas and coffees as well as from caffeinated brews for the first six weeks. Why? As usual, there's a psychological as well as physiological reason.

From the psychological standpoint, if you switch from caffeinated coffee or tea to a decaffeinated beverage, you're not really changing your habit. You're not going through any of the changes in attitude and behavior that promise a permanent change. You're not avoiding any of the triggers that established your habit in the first place. In some ways, it could be said that you're fooling yourself. You're still getting the same taste and wishing for the same old jolt. People who switch to "decaf" often find that within a few days they're back on the caffeinated beverage. When you haven't made a genuine, deliberate behavioral change, the step between a cup of decaf and a cup of full-strength coffee or tea is just too short. Decaf is like methadone; it substitutes a new set of problems for the old, and doesn't really help the user to beat his addiction.

The biochemical reasons for avoiding decaffeinated beverages are really more compelling than the psychological ones. The fact that coffee or tea is decaffeinated doesn't eliminate all its physical dangers. For example, you can be allergic to the coffee beans themselves; decaffeinating the beans doesn't eliminate the allergens. If you're allergic, you'll continue to suffer from any of the symptoms that regular coffee may have caused: headache, diarrhea, constipation, mood swings, and nausea. On a more serious level, decaffeinated coffee and tea have been linked to many of the same diseases connected with caffeine, including pancreatic cancer, myocardial infarction, and fibrocystic breast disease.

I do believe that if after six weeks you begin to have an occasional cup of coffee or tea, you're better off having a decaffeinated kind because you'll be avoiding some of the problems created by caffeine. But for the first six weeks, and certainly for the extent of the Medical Makeover, avoid all coffees and teas.

What Do I Drink Instead?

The very best substitute for coffee and tea is herbal tea, and most of my patients have become connoisseurs. Fortunately, there are many kinds of herbal tea on the market these days, and they're easy to find. Even the major tea manufacturers, recognizing their popularity, have come out with herbal teas. I remember one of my patients—who drank up to seven cups of coffee a day—telling me that she could never imagine drinking herbal tea; it seemed like a wimpy thing to do, and she had always felt impatient when someone in a restaurant ordered just a cup of hot water at the end of the meal and produced an herbal tea bag. I was amused by the strength of her feelings and hoped she would be able to kick her caffeine habit despite them. Sure enough, within a few days of giving up coffee she had joined the ranks of those who order "just a cup of hot water" at the end of restaurant meals, and is now as messianic as an ex-smoker about the dangers of caffeine and the virtues of herbal tea.

Two other drinks, Pero and Postum, are popular with some people as substitutes for coffee, and they may be worth a try. Both are made from grain and are available in health food stores. Whatever you substitute for a morning or evening or coffee-break drink, it's important that you drink it unsweetened. Next week you're going to be working on sugar, and if you develop the habit of drinking five cups of herb tea with five teaspoons of sugar or honey per day, you'll be working against yourself. There's no point in acquiring a taste for sweet herb tea one week only to have to eliminate it the next. So right from the beginning, drink these substitute beverages plain, without sugar, honey, or sugar substitutes. You can, however, add a slice of lemon or orange or even a small bit of fruit juice if you like.

If you're accustomed to drinking carbonated beverages, with or without caffeine, this is the week to stop. Many kinds contain caffeine, but even if your favorite brand doesn't, it's still not doing you any good. If you drink sweetened soda, you're getting up to six teaspoons of sugar in every eight-ounce serving! If you drink the artificially sweetened kind, you're dependent on that sweet taste, and you may be at risk because of the sweetener itself. As long as you're going to be working on sugar next week, begin now by stocking up on substitutes for carbonated beverages. When you buy your herb tea, pick up some club soda or seltzer, or a soda siphon so you can make your own seltzer. Mix the seltzer with a dash of fruit juice, or add a slice of orange or lemon for a refreshing, flavorful healthy substitute for a can of soda.

Buy these beverages before you begin your caffeine-free week. The preparation itself will commit you to making the change. If you find yourself on a cold morning with no herbal tea or other substitute, and there's a can of coffee staring you in the face, you'll find it difficult to resist.

Plan in Advance

It's best to have a few days to plan and prepare before you begin your anticaffeine campaign. From a practical standpoint, it's much better to start on a Saturday if you work a normal work week. That's because you'll have two days at home to recover from any withdrawal symptoms. You can also plan your time so that you can avoid doing demanding work if you're suffering from withdrawal headaches. Finally, you'll avoid the situations that you've come to associate with caffeine: the morning coffee break, the afternoon cola or chocolate bar, the bedtime cocoa or tea. (If you don't work a Monday-to-Friday week, quit caffeine on the beginning of one of your days off from work.) I've heard it suggested that you can try to give up caffeine while on vacation, but again, in my experience, this isn't an effective approach. If you're not working, you may be more painfully aware of caffeine-withdrawal symptoms, and I can't think of a more unpleasant way to spend a vacation than withdrawing from an addiction. A regular or perhaps a three-day weekend should be enough to get you over the worst of your withdrawal symptoms.

Analyze Your Triggers

Every addiction has triggers that will spur you to indulge—people, places, things, or events which you associate with the addiction and make it difficult to avoid it. In order to kick caffeine successfully, you need to recognize what triggers encourage you to use it. This might seem like a meaningless exercise at first. After all, you may tell yourself, I'll just give it up and that will be that. But if you take this approach, you'll probably find yourself in a situation where you have to make an on-the-spot decision, and these moments are the most dangerous kind.

Take a few minutes and think of each time you have a cup of coffee or tea or a drink of cola, or even a chocolate bar if you eat one regularly. What time of day is it? Are you alone? Do you tend to drink coffee before a meeting, during a meeting, just during coffee breaks, after meals? Do you have a chocolate bar as a reward in the middle of the afternoon? Do you begin the day by having coffee or tea with your spouse and/or end it the same way? Make a quick list of all your triggers.

Once you know the triggers, decide how you're going to avoid them. If you usually have coffee or tea in restaurants, tuck some herbal tea bags in your pocket as substitutes. If you want to join your colleagues in an afternoon coffee break, make sure herbal tea is in your desk. If you are used to having a chocolate bar in the afternoon, have a piece of fruit each day instead. Pam H., one of my patients, was tempted by certain cappuccino cafés she passed on her way to and from the office. She had always enjoyed stopping in for a coffee break, and had fond associations with that experience. She found that she was much better off changing her route to work. If she didn't smell the coffee and cinnamon, she didn't miss it; if she had to pass the café twice a day, she felt sorely tempted to go in. Sometimes it's easier to avoid a trigger altogether.

If you're used to having a cup of coffee and a cigarette to start your day, let me remind you that nicotine doubles the rate at which your body metabolizes caffeine:

Smoking can make you want to drink more coffee. At the end of the Medical Makeover, you're going to give up smoking; for now, make sure you have a coffee substitute on hand if you can't resist a cigarette.

The point of recognizing your triggers is that you can plan ahead and avoid spontaneous decisions at times when your willpower may be weak. Plan this, your first week, in advance, taking into account all the triggers that you're likely to encounter. Make decisions on which ones you can handle by using substitutes and which ones you should avoid. Make sure that your substitutes are on hand when you need them.

Recruit Your Helpers

You'll find your Makeover is much easier at every point of the way if you recruit helpers. This book should serve as a major helper. If you feel your resolve on caffeine weakening, for example, go back and read the beginning of this chapter and remind yourself of all the damage that caffeine is doing to your body. Don't forget to pay attention to how you feel when you drink caffeine and how you begin to feel when you give it up. That memory alone should stiffen your resolve.

Enlist the people in your life to help you give up caffeine. Explain to your colleagues at work that you can't consume any caffeine. Tell them you've developed an allergy to it. You can also use that excuse in restaurants. If your spouse drinks coffee or tea, perhaps you can convince him or her to join you in abstaining. Many of my patients have told me that though they begin the Medical Makeover alone, their spouses often join them when they see the results their mates are enjoying. It's much easier to begin the day with herbal tea, especially the first week, if you don't have someone across the table from you drinking coffee. But even if your spouse won't join you, explain why you're giving up caffeine and ask him or her to be supportive.

Caffeine Withdrawal

If you ever doubted that caffeine was an addiction, all doubts will be erased when you experience withdrawal. Most of my patients have been amazed at the way their bodies react when they give up caffeine, because they never suspected it had had such a powerful hold on them.

If you quit caffeine on a Saturday morning, your most likely symptom will be a feeling of lethargy in the early part of the day, followed by a headache in the afternoon. The headache may last from three to six hours, though in some cases it can last even longer. It may be intensified by bending over. Napping and/or lying down can make the headache worse. My patients also report increased irritability, inability to work effectively, and restlessness. Unfortunately, I can't recommend any pain reliever that will successfully treat the headache except those containing caffeine, and of course those are the last things you want to take. Aspirin, however, doesn't contain caffeine and it may help you. In addition to a headache, you may also feel general fatigue, nausea and, sometimes, vomiting, depression, and an overpowering urge to yawn.

Michael M., who had a severe caffeine addiction, felt so awful when he gave up caffeine that he asked his wife and child to leave him alone for the entire weekend. Fortunately, they visited her mother who lived nearby, and when they returned Michael was human again. He told me that he was completely shocked by his reaction, and that if he hadn't been told what to expect, he would have been terribly concerned about his health. He wound up going to bed for the entire weekend, and he says that it took him almost a full week to feel completely recovered. Of course, this is an extreme case, but countless patients have called me in the middle of their caffeine withdrawal, concerned about what's happening to them. You can see why it's best to quit on a weekend so you don't have to cope with withdrawal effects and the demands of work at the same time.

Keeping on Track

Once you've gone through caffeine withdrawal, the worst is over. There are two things, however, I suggest you do throughout the week to keep yourself on track.

1. *Pay Attention to How You Feel*. This is important. Most of us are so busy with work and recreation and the details of our lives that we pay little attention to how we actually feel. In the course of the Medical Makeover, it's crucial that you develop the habit of noticing how you feel. Then, as you eliminate your bad habits, you'll get the positive reinforcement of feeling better as a reward, and you'll be aware of your newly achieved vitality.

Begin this habit the first week. Notice how withdrawal feels. Notice how you feel at the end of the first two days. Do you have more energy? Fewer headaches? Do you sleep better? Wake up more alert? Pay attention so you can appreciate the progress you're making and stick to the Makeover.

2. *Talk to Yourself*. I do this all the time, and I encourage my patients to do it too. Tell yourself that you're making progress. Remind yourself that you're feeling better. Remind yourself that you're moving closer to your goal. Talk to yourself throughout the day about how you're going to avoid triggers and make substitutes. Monitoring yourself in this way can be very beneficial and can get you over some rough periods.

Dealing with Relapse

If you do break down and have caffeine at some point in the Medical Makeover, all will not be lost. As I said before, after six weeks you can reintroduce a small amount of caffeine into your diet with no serious ill effects. If you do so, I think it's best to make it at least a partially decaffeinated beverage. Some of my patients treat themselves to a cup of half-regular half-decaffeinated coffee on weekends with no harm done. The danger with doing this is that your habit can come back. Somehow it's easier to go from having a weekend coffee to a daily coffee than to go from nothing to a daily coffee.

If you do have a relapse, take it in stride and don't be discouraged. I sometimes give my body a test if I go back to a bit of sugar or caffeine. I pay careful attention to how these things make me feel, and decide all over again that the brief pleasure isn't worth the aftereffects. If you do have some caffeine, notice how it affects you, not just immediately but also that evening and the next morning. That way your relapse won't be wasted; abstaining totally can be a device to strengthen your resolve.

Remember also that you will be taking the antioxidants I suggested to prepare you biochemically to give up coffee. And it won't be impossible to quit, no matter how much you rely on it, no matter how many cups a day you drink.

Week Two: Sugar

How's this for a recipe: Take a large glass of water, add some artificial coloring and flavoring, and twelve tea spoons of sugar. Stir and drink. Have one of these drinks with lunch, in the afternoon, after work, after exercising, and while you watch TV. By the end of the day you will have consumed sixty teaspoons of sugar.

No doubt you think this recipe sounds impossible, but in fact it's a broad outline of the ingredients used in popular soft drinks. They're really little more than sugar and water. And even if you never drink sugar-sweetened soft drinks, you probably consume far more sugar than you should. Most Americans consume between 100 and 128 pounds per year. If you know what a one-pound box of sugar looks like, imagine eating one third of the box every day. That's about how much sugar you eat even if you rarely use the sugar bowl. Where does all this sugar come from? It is by far the most common food additive in our diets. It is even more common than salt. If, for example, you put a tablespoon of ketchup on your hamburger, you're adding a teaspoon of sugar. Even your low-fat fruit yogurt has about seven and a half teaspoons of sugar in it.

Most people recognize that sugar isn't particularly good for them, but they're not certain why. One of my patients, Susan K., a thirty-year-old woman who works on Wall Street, told me that she drank up to six cups of coffee every day with two or three teaspoons of sugar in each cup. She also had a few soft drinks during the day and an occasional candy bar. Susan was suffering from severe headaches and afternoon fatigue. When I pointed out to her the extremely high amount of sugar she was eating every day, her expression was sheepish. She thought that she probably ate too much sugar, but explained that she didn't think it was really a problem because she wasn't overweight. This is a typical misconception about sugar. So many of my patients believe that the real danger of sugar is weight gain.

While the excess calories in sugar are definitely a health hazard, they are not the most serious effect of excess sugar consumption. The sugar in your diet, in addition to contributing to overweight, has a range of short- and long-term adverse effects on your health that are much more subtle and pervasive. I've found that excess sugar consumption is a major factor in many of the health problems that bring my patients to see me. It contributes to their headaches, fatigue, irritability, inability to concentrate, and it makes dieting more difficult. Sugar also does damage beyond the effect it alone has on your body. It reinforces your other bad health habits and amplifies their adverse effects.

This Week's Goal

In this, the second week of the Makeover, your goal is to eliminate sugar from your diet. Because you've already given up caffeine, you probably noticed that you're not feeling the extreme highs and lows that you may have experienced before. But because sugar has such a powerful effect on your metabolism, it won't be until the end of this second week that the benefits of your Makeover begin to become dramatically apparent.

Some of my patients have claimed to have a powerful sweet tooth and couldn't imagine life without sugar. A few patients have actually had problems with sweet binges, in which they would lose control and eat an entire large bag of candy or a pint or two of ice cream. These people anticipated that giving up sugar would be the most difficult week of the Makeover for them. But again, giving up sugar isn't just a matter of willpower; if you've got a sweeth tooth, it's not because you're a weak person. More likely it's a manifestation of your particular biochemistry. With the proper supplements—especially one called chromium, or glucose tolerance factor, that my patients have found enormously helpful—you'll discover that your sweet tooth can be conquered.

The biggest challenge of the second week will be to learn to recognize the hidden sources of sugar in your diet so that you can eliminate them.

Sweet Seduction

While many of us love sugar, we don't take it seriously as a food. Sugary things are usually considered a treat or a reward—no dessert if you don't finish your vegetables! Even as adults we have a curiously ambivalent attitude toward sugar. We think of it as a childish food, but we can't resist it. The seriousness with which restaurant-goers consider their entrée orders dissolves in the face of the dessert cart. There's usually at least one smirk or guilty giggle as the waiter tries to tempt us into breaking down and trying the Sinful Chocolate Surprise. Just notice how often adjectives like "sinful," "wicked," and "decadent" are used to describe a dessert.

If sweets are really so sinful, wicked, and decadent, why do we eat so many of them? For one thing, like caffeine, sugar is an *acceptable* addiction. It's socially acceptable to talk about your chocolate addiction, or your occasional Twinkie binge, or your uncontrollable lust for ice cream. In some instances it's even a deliberate ploy: I once read about a very thin woman who recommended that other slender people be sure to order dessert when having a business lunch or dinner. Like a dog lying on its back to indicate submission, ordering dessert keeps the other party from hating you for being thin.

The proliferation of "gourmet" ice creams, chocolate chip cookies, and imported-chocolate shops in all major cities is an indication of how sugar has become an acceptable treat for adults who are otherwise sophisticated about health and nutrition. I've noticed that many of my patients may be scrupulous about working out four or five times a week or running regularly, but because of their regular exercise they think that eating sweets is an indulgence they can afford. This attitude grows out of the misconception that if you're not fat, you can eat anything you want.

Most people begin a love affair with sugar shortly after birth. It's been common practice for many hospitals to give bottles with sugar water to newborns on the theory that if the baby has any sucking problems, the hospital will be able to discover them early by noting how the baby takes the sugar-water bottle. From that first taste on, many of us are hooked. We grew up on heavily sweetened breakfast cereals, sugary soda pop, and candy. We've grown so accustomed to sweet foods that we don't even notice that sugar is a significant ingredient in such things as spaghetti sauce, bouillon cubes, salad dressings, and even soups and cured meats.

Is there any natural reason for our yearning for sweets? Some researchers postulate that at one point in our evolution, a taste for sweets was an important instinct. Before man perfected his ability to acquire food through hunting, he depended on what he could gather from the forest floor for nutrition. If he ate anything he could put his hands on, he would probably have consumed mainly cellulose, which is indigestible and nutritionally not very valuable. But if he depended on eating things that were sweet, this would have been a more reliable guide to selecting foods that provided the calories he needed for energy. Obviously, a taste for sweets is, like the fight-or-flight reaction to stress, an evolutionary anachronism. In a modern world where sugar is a cheap, plentiful food additive, a sweet tooth is not only anachronistic, it's dangerous.

Do We Need Any Sugar?

Does sugar have *any* value in the diet? Not really. Not in its most popular form of common table sugar.

Our bodies derive energy from three sources: carbohydrates, fats, and proteins. Carbohydrates are our bodies' main source of energy. They provide calories for energy by producing heat in the body, and they help to regulate the metabolism of fats and proteins. The three principal carbohydrates in foods are sugars, starches, and cellulose. Cellulose, which we commonly think of as fiber, doesn't contribute much energy value, but it does provide bulk. Starches give us a steady source of energy as our bodies break them down into simple sugars, some to be used immediately and some to be stored for future use. Sugars, like those present in table sugars or honey, are quickly digested and give an immediate boost of energy. But that boost takes its toll on the body in other ways; in fact, we can get all the energy we need, and far more efficiently, from the steady burning of starch.

The body does need glucose—one of the components of sugar—to function. The brain in particular depends on a steady supply of glucose. But the body can readily obtain all the glucose it needs from the breakdown of complex carbohydrates found in fruits, vegetables, and whole grains. We need about 75 grams of glucose daily, and can readily obtain this amount from just one meal that includes pasta, broccoli, bread, and a fruit dessert.

In comparing how the body uses starch versus how it uses sugar, I think of a driving habit of a friend. He pumps the gas pedal constantly, gunning the motor so the car will surge forward for a distance, then taking his foot off the pedal until the car glides to a near halt. He takes advantage of every hill to gain speed, and will let that speed carry the car almost to a stop before hitting the gas pedal again. His erratic acceleration is literally sickening, and I'm convinced that he winds up using more gas than if he kept the car at a steady speed. Sugar has a similar effect on the body as an erratic foot on the gas pedal. It jolts you forward and then slows you down. It's not coincidental that the effects of this stop-start method of energy supply are similar to car sickness: When your energy drops, you can feel dizzy, fatigued, sleepy, and light-headed. Complex carbohydrates, on the other hand, give you a steady supply of forward motion. They are a far preferable source of energy.

Sugar: The Nutritional Blank

If it were just a matter of sugar being a less efficient energy source than starch, you could probably accept it as a reasonable alternative to starch and let it go at that. But there are more serious problems with sugar consumption.

For one thing, eating sugar is like firing a nutritional blank. It doesn't make enough of a contribution to your dietary needs, and it crowds out other, more valuable foods. It has been estimated that the average American consumes 24 percent of his or her calories in sugar daily. Subtracting the portion of this percentage that comes from natural sugars in dairy products, fruits, and vegetables, we find that 18 percent of the calories comes directly from table sugar. Nearly one fifth of your daily calories come from a source that doesn't have enough nutritional value to carry its weight.

If we take the total amount of sugar in our diet—24 percent—and add to it the average amount of fat we consume daily—35 percent—we can see that most of us are eating a diet in which nearly 60 percent of the caloric intake comes from sugar and fat. As both sugar and fat offer little in the way of nutritional value, we depend on the remaining 40 percent of our diet to get the nutrients we need for health. Obviously, we are not likely to accomplish this feat. Over the long haul such suboptimum nutrition can result in borderline malnutrition, and is responsible for the kind of daily adverse effects that my patients complain of, such as fatigue, headaches, and irritability.

Sugar and Heart Disease

In addition to making you fat, encouraging you to overeat, stressing your body on a secret, daily basis, and giving you vague nagging symptoms, sugar is contributing to future chronic disease.

Sugar has been implicated in the development of heart disease, the leading cause of death and disability in this country. Studies by Dr. John Yudkin, professor of nutrition and dietetics at the University of London, indicate that someone who eats four ounces of sugar daily has more than five times the chance of developing heart disease than someone eating only half as much sugar. In a recent study done by the U.S. Department of Agriculture's Nutrition Institute in Beltsville, Maryland, two groups of people were put on similar diets except that one group received 30 percent of its calories from sugar and the other group received 30 percent from starch. The people on the sugar diet developed high levels of blood fats (cholesterol and triglycerides), which promote the development of heart disease. It also seems that some people—about fifty million Americans—are carbohydrate sensitive, and have a genetic predisposition to developing high levels of triglycerides if they eat a great deal of sugar. These people are at higher risk for developing heart disease.

Additionally, it's well known that obese people are at greater risk for developing heart disease, and large amounts of sugar in the diet are closely linked with obesity. While there is still more research to be done on the subject, there's no question that too much sugar in your diet will make it more likely that you'll develop heart disease.

Diabetes: Our Sixth Leading Killer

Diabetes mellitus is the sixth leading cause of death in the United States. Serious on its own terms, diabetes is also a risk factor for heart disease, our number one killer. Studies have shown that people who have diabetes develop heart disease more often, more seriously, and more prematurely than non-diabetics.

We've known for a long time that there is a link between sugar consumption and diabetes, but now there are two theories on how sugar contributes to the development of the disease. Diabetes, or hyperglycemia, is—like hypoglycemia, or low blood sugar—a manifestation of your body's inability to control the level of sugar in the blood. Normally insulin, which is produced by the pancreas, transports sugar from the blood into the cells of the body.

But in a person suffering from diabetes, either the pancreas can no longer supply sufficient insulin or the body loses its sensitivity to insulin, and the sugar in the blood rises to dangerous levels. There is a genetic tendency toward diabetes. It has been speculated that more than 20 percent of the population suffers from this tendency. If you have a family history of diabetes, this second week of the Medical Makeover may be one of the most important weeks, as it could help you avoid a serious chronic disease.

Even people who don't have a genetic tendency toward diabetes can't ignore the connection between sugar and diabetes. Research has demonstrated that, over a period of time, a diet high in sugar may wear out the pancreas so that it can no longer supply the necessary insulin. While your pancreas will normally effectively produce insulin throughout your lifetime, if you eat large quantities of sugar, the pancreas could become exhausted after fifty years. That's a possible explanation for why so many older people develop diabetes: A lifetime of overconsumption of sugar has caught up with them.

Sugar and Your Teeth and Bones

Most of my patients don't seem to be very interested in the fact that too much sugar causes cavities. They feel they're beyond that stage in their lives. But the patients who do eat a lot of sugar are often troubled by cavities. When those cavities begin to appear between the front teeth and become cosmetic problems, and when teeth eroded by years of decay begin to require complicated and expensive dental work, these patients begin to take a more serious attitude toward the effect of sugar on their teeth.

Sugar doesn't cause tooth decay but it promotes it. It allows a bacterium normally present in the mouth to produce an acid that eats away at tooth enamel. Obviously, cutting sugar out of your diet will have a beneficial effect on your teeth. I remember one delighted patient who routinely had one or two cavities a year announcing that she had had her first cavity-free dental checkup in years after giving up sugar. She was more pleased about her weight loss, but even though her medical plan didn't cover dental care, she now had a little extra money each year she could spend on her new, smaller-size wardrobe.

Sugar attacks more than teeth. It's a factor in the development of osteoporosis, the weakening of bones that affects so many older women. Sugar decreases the amount of phosphorus in the blood to such a degree that for two to five hours after a sugar snack, the body can't sustain calcification. If you eat sweets a few times a day, during most of your waking hours sugar is contributing to the deterioration of your bones. In addition, sugar depletes calcium, a mineral that is deficient in many women. Large amounts of calcium have been found in urine after consumption of a sugar-rich meal. If the drain of calcium and phosphorus is great enough, heart disturbances are possible.

Low Blood Sugar and the Medical Makeover

A number of years ago articles began to appear in the popular press about low blood sugar, also called hypoglycemia. Paradoxically, hypoglycemia can be caused by eating too much sugar. When the sugar reaches the blood, which happens within seconds after you eat it, the body produces insulin to normalize the blood-sugar level. In a person suffering from hypoglycemia, the body may produce too much insulin. The blood-sugar level is decreased so rapidly and thoroughly that the person suffers distressing symptoms.

The symptoms of hypoglycemia include headaches,

fatigue, depression, anxiety, dizziness, lack of mental alertness, and rapid mood swings. People began flocking to their doctors to be treated for blood-sugar problems because so many suffered from one or more of these symptoms. Many of my patients at that time came to be treated for low blood sugar. A few years went by and the medical establishment, recognizing that low blood sugar had become a "medical fad," argued that there was no such thing as hypoglycemia. We went from witnessing a plague of hypoglycemia to a complete dismissal of the disorder.

The truth lies somewhere in between. I am convinced that while it may be true that very few people can be diagnosed by means of the accepted glucose-tolerance test as classic cases of hypoglycemia, large numbers of people have some difficulty in handling refined sugar in their diet, which gives them the common symptoms of fatigue, inability to concentrate, etc., that we have been discussing.

In my practice I see many people with blood-sugar problems. They have periods when they feel tired, weak, irritable, moody, headachy, and depressed. Many of them have been to other doctors and have had all the routine blood tests and were told that there was nothing wrong with them, that they had no definite medical problem. But they knew that something was wrong, and they were convinced that it wasn't all in their minds. I gave these patients the standard test for hypoglycemia because their symptoms were classic for that condition. This test, the glucose tolerance test, is administered over a period of hours. It measures the level of sugar in the blood after the patient has consumed a large sugar load. The sugar load may re-create the distressing symptoms peculiar to hypoglycemia. But the diagnosis is made on the basis of standard numbers: A sugar level below a certain arbitrary percentage, in conjunction with the symptoms, determines if the patient has hypoglycemia.

But I began to notice a curious thing: Though many of my patients didn't have the classic low blood-sugar values on the glucose tolerance test, they did experience their troublesome symptoms during the test, and each person had these symptoms at different blood-sugar levels. So some people's blood-sugar level could be far above that which would be considered a "low" level and still suffer low blood-sugar symptoms. According to the standard test guidelines, they weren't suffering from hypoglycemia. But I found that when I treated them as if they had hypoglycemia—by working with them on diet and giving them vitamin-mineral supplements—they improved and their symptoms almost always disappeared.

As I began to research the latest findings on hypoglycemia, I discovered that the condition is not as simple as was first believed, and many people may suffer from it to a greater or lesser degree. If they do not suffer from classic hypoglycemia, they do have vague symptoms that are exacerbated by eating too much sugar.

The Stress of Sugar

Just as caffeine is an addiction, so is a craving for sugar. My patients who tell me they have a sweet tooth report symptoms common to all addictions: increased consumption of the substance over a period of time, withdrawal symptoms when it is denied, and intense cravings for it. But with the program that has worked with my patients—many of whom had said they could never give up their sweets—you won't experience withdrawal and you won't crave sugar anymore. And you will feel better. That's a promise.

Sugar does give you a temporary lift, but over the long haul it puts the body under major stress. When you eat too much of it, refined or otherwise, the blood-sugar level rises to abnormal heights. The body tries to get everything to return to normal by having the pancreas produce insulin, the hormone which regulates sugar levels in the blood. If you're not a sugar addict, your pancreas can easily handle isolated doses of sugar. But many of us, whether we know it or not, have become sugar addicts. So when you eat that candy bar—which contains more sugar than you need for a week—up goes your blood-sugar level, your pancreas kicks on, and what does it do? Paradoxically, it overreacts and produces too much insulin. It's no longer a good regulatory organ. This flood of insulin in the bloodstream makes your blood-sugar level take a nose dive. In response, the adrenal glands release antistress hormones which in turn release the sugar that is stored in the liver for emergencies. The net result? Everything gets worn out—the pancreas, the adrenal glands, and the liver. And you don't feel so good. It's as if you're on a sort of yo-yo.

First, you get a spurt of energy from the candy bar. But that doesn't last very long. Your insulin level rises and your spirits fall. Suddenly you feel tired, irritable, moody, depressed, and you don't know why. But then the adrenal glands start working and you experience feelings associated with anxiety: nervousness, palpitations, butterflies in the stomach.

Most people don't attribute these feelings to the candy bar they had an hour ago; they think that it's the cranky child, the checks that didn't come, a tough day at the office, a flat tire that causes them. But when your blood-sugar level remains on a more even keel, you're better able to weather the stress storms that come your way. You're biochemically shipshape.

The repeated ingestion of sugar, with the resultant biochemical stress reactions, contributes heavily to feeling run down. You're no longer able to produce the required amounts of antistress hormones that allow you to maintain a state of well-being and homeostasis. When my patients reach this second stage of the blood-sugar problem, they complain of a chronic irritability and a chronic sense of fatigue, unrelieved by sleep. By this time, they notice they cannot go very long without eating or their symptoms increase. In a normal person, who isn't operating at crisis level because of blood-sugar fluctuations, the body maintains its blood-sugar level by releasing antistress hormones, which in turn release glycogen from the liver at a steady pace; and while you might feel hungry, you won't lose your temper over little things. When you're run down, the body cannot maintain biochemical or emotional tranquillity, and lack of food can put you in a tailspin. Given all that, it's not hard to understand how sugar can become an addiction as you try to avoid those symptoms. You want a sugar fix.

Sugar, Stress, and Overweight

It is easy to see how sugar addiction leads to weight gain. While two after-dinner mints may have the same total calories as a fresh apple, the apple will make you feel much fuller. You'll probably eat nearly a dozen after-dinner mints before you begin to feel as full as you would after eating the apple. Most sweet things are giving you too many calories for the bulk and not filling you up. Moreover, as far as overall nutrition is concerned, you're filling up on useless calories.

While most of us know that there's a direct relationship between sugar and overweight, we're not familiar with the indirect relationship between the two.

Recent research has come up with some startling news: Insulin affects the brain as profoundly as it does the body. Dr. Judith Rodin, professor of psychology and psychiatry at Yale University, found that high insulin levels make you more hungry, make you eat more, and make sweets taste better.

"Insulin, in fact, appears to have much more to do

with appetite than your level of blood sugar does," she wrote recently in *American Health*. She was reporting on an extensive study that clearly demonstrated that when men and women were pumped with insulin, "they became hungrier and liked sweet tastes more." The experiment may explain why some diabetics who receive large amounts of insulin complain that they're hungry all the time.

What these findings mean to you is that eating sugar can stimulate a vicious circle: The more you eat, the more you want to eat. Eliminate sugar, particularly the kind used in most baked goods and prepared foods, and it will be much easier to control your appetite.

As a bonus, your overall nutrition will be improved. Your blood-sugar levels won't shoot up and down erratically, and you won't crave sugar to "control" the highs and lows that result from eating sweets. The end result of eliminating sugar from your diet? If you're overweight, you will probably shed some pounds.

The Step-by-Step Approach

As with coffee, if you try to stop eating sugar without help, you will usually fail. If you have been consuming large amounts of sugar, your body has become dependent on it. You find it difficult to cope without sugar. But, as with coffee, I won't let you go cold turkey without biochemical help.

There are three things that will help you give up sugar no matter how powerful your sweet tooth. All three have to do with changing your body chemistry so that your blood sugar is kept on a more even keel. Not only will this help you fight the urge to binge, it will generally improve your energy level, your moods, and your sense of well-being. The three things are:

1. The supplement chromium
2. The glycemic index
3. Regular meals at regular times

Chromium Supplement

Many of my patients have come to think of chromium as a "wonder pill." It's not, of course. It's a mineral supplement and its importance in our diet began to be recognized in the 1950s. The reason my patients are such fans of chromium is that it has a very dramatic effect on their metabolism, particularly if they have strong sugar cravings.

Chromium first drew attention when it was discovered that it improved glucose intolerance in rats. (Glucose intolerance refers to the inability to metabolize sugar effectively, resulting in energy highs and lows.) Rats who were given brewers' yeast, a rich source of chromium, were better able to utilize sugar for energy. It was finally discovered that a substance named glucose tolerance factor (GTF), a form of chromium, was helping the rats. Not only did the glucose-intolerant rats suffer from chromium deficiency, but their growth was impaired and they had elevated blood cholesterol, fatty deposits in their arteries, a decreased life span, and decreased fertility. We now know that chromium is an essential trace element for man as well as rats.

Though only two people have been discovered to have a serious chromium deficiency since 1977, research shows that most Americans have a marginal deficiency. It isn't enough to provoke severe symptoms. But for those people who are prone to blood-sugar control problems, this deficiency is enough to affect their metabolism in ways that could create subtle symptoms and damage long-term health.

The average person needs to absorb only 1 microgram

of chromium from food each day. Chromium is available in small amounts in such foods as fish, poultry, meats, whole-grain breads and cereals, cheese, nuts, dried fruits, and certain vegetables, and you would think that someone on an average diet would have no trouble getting this daily microgram. Unfortunately, our bodies seem to be able to absorb only 1 to 2 percent of the mineral from foods. Therefore, to get your single microgram, you would have to eat between 50 and 100 micrograms daily, and the average person eats only 33 micrograms each day.

Some people are at greater risk of chromium loss. Those who are under a great deal of stress, pregnant or breast-feeding women, and people who are regular, heavy exercisers—runners, for example—are often deficient in chromium. Moreover, people who drink coffee or tea or eat a lot of sugar often have depleted stores of chromium. This means that people who have a sweet tooth are often the least able to metabolize sugar effectively because of insufficient chromium stores. This may be why some of my patients who have strong sweet cravings seem to receive the most benefit from the chromium supplement.

Brewers' yeast is the best source of chromium from foods. It contains between 6 and 60 micrograms per tablespoon. There is now on the market an enriched yeast that has more available chromium in it; it's a better source than regular brewers' yeast. If you can find this kind of yeast and the taste is agreeable to you, fine. But in my experience, a chromium supplement in pill form is simpler and more palatable. However, it's important to get the right kind. I experimented with different kinds and dosages and met with little success until I found a chromium supplement that is readily absorbed by the body. I discovered that the trivalent form of chromium in dosages of 100 micrograms taken three times a day before meals is most effective for controlling sweet cravings, reducing appetite, and keeping energy levels up between meals.

My patients reported good results both in controlling their sweet cravings and in diminishing their vague symptoms.

Now I don't claim that a chromium imbalance or deficiency per se is the sole cause of a blood-sugar problem. But I know from experience that a chromium supplement can make a significant difference. I think that with the right diet—no sugar and eating regular meals at regular times—you can control your sweet tooth and the vague symptoms of blood-sugar problems. But with the right diet plus the chromium supplement, you can also *cure* those symptoms.

The Glycemic Index

Just as sugar makes you crave more of it, certain foods we think of as innocent have the same ability. These foods, as seemingly benign as white potatoes, quickly boost blood sugar and, accordingly, insulin levels. Consequently, they make you hungry and likely to eat more.

When researchers at the University of Toronto tested various carbohydrate foods, they found wide—and surprising—variance in how quickly and how intensely blood-sugar levels rose after the foods were eaten. These foods have now been charted according to their glycemic index, which is a measure of the speed and intensity of the blood-glucose response after the food is eaten. A food with a high *glycemic index* is a fast releaser, and should be avoided when trying to control blood sugar. Slow releasers, on the other hand, bring only moderate changes in blood sugar and have a low glycemic index.

What foods can be biochemically troublesome? Carrots and parsnips. Beets have more effect on blood sugar than pastry or a bowl of ice cream. Of all the complex carbohydrates tested, peanuts, cooked dried peas and beans, oatmeal, and pasta had the least effect on blood sugar.

The following chart lists the glycemic index for a number of carbohydrate foods. Slow releasers, which bring only moderate changes in blood sugar, have a low glycemic index. In each group shown here, slow releasers are listed first. For the duration of the Medical Makeover, try to avoid eating those foods with a high glycemic index number. While you don't need to abstain from, say, peas, you should limit your consumption of this vegetable to no more than once a week. And carrots, a food with a very high glycemic index, should certainly not be eaten alone as a snack. Don't take a bag of carrot sticks to the office to munch on! If you have a choice between a sweet potato and a white potato, choose the sweet potato. Oatmeal makes a much better breakfast than cornflakes, even if you do manage to find a brand without sugar in it.

Use the glycemic index with common sense. Try to avoid the highly rated foods, and always choose in favor of bulk and fiber. For example, an apple is a better snack than raisins.

Honey and Sugars		Breakfast Cereals	
Fructose	20	Oatmeal	49
Sucrose	59	All-Bran	51
Honey	87	Swiss muesli	66
Glucose	100	Shredded wheat	67
		Cornflakes	80
Bread, Pasta, Corn, and Rice			
Whole-wheat spaghetti	42	**Fruits**	
White spaghetti	50	Apples (Golden Delicious)	39
Sweet corn	59	Oranges	40
Brown rice	66	Orange juice	46
White bread	69	Bananas	62
Whole-wheat bread	72	Raisins	64
White rice	72		

Root Vegetables		Lentils	29
Sweet potatoes	48	Kidney beans	29
Yams	51	Black-eyed peas	33
Beets	64	Chickpeas	36
White potatoes	70	Lima beans	36
Instant mashed potatoes	80	Canned baked beans	40
Carrots	92	Frozen peas	51
Parsnips	97		
		Odds and Ends	
Dairy Products		Peanuts	13
Skim milk	32	Sausages	28
Whole milk	34	Fish sticks	38
Ice cream	36	Tomato soup	38
Yogurt	36	Sponge cake	46
Peas and Beans (Dried, Canned, Frozen)			
Soybeans	15		

Regular Meals at Regular Times

Next week we're going to work on nutrition in earnest. But in order to help your body adjust readily to the elimination of sugar there's one diet-related thing you have to do this week: You must eat regular meals at regular times each day. You must eat breakfast, lunch, and dinner—it's absolutely crucial that you do so. Many of my patients skip breakfast entirely or have just coffee and a doughnut, and lunch is something like yogurt, eaten at the desk. By dinnertime, or even late afternoon, they're starving, and that's when they consume the bulk of the day's calories. But since they're always vulnerable to snacking, they often have sweet snacks two or three times a day. Once they make a point of eating three regular meals, it's much easier to feel in charge of what they eat rather than being driven by ravenous hunger once or twice a day. They also enjoy a more consistent energy level throughout the day.

At this point you don't have to fuss about precisely what you're eating as long as it's a reasonable amount and doesn't have sugar in it. But don't skip any of the three meals. If you do, your blood sugar will plunge, and you'll want to have a sugar snack. Your body will yearn for the quick-energy boost of a sugar load. And remember that when your blood sugar is low, your mood and certainly your willpower are affected. It's the worst possible time to have to make a decision about what sort of snack to have.

You can have snacks. In fact, if you're used to having something sweet at coffee break, it's a good idea to use a substitute. Last week you gave up caffeine but found substitutes so you wouldn't have to change your behavior completely. It should be the same with sugar. A piece of fruit makes a perfect snack.

The idea is to eat foods that will be digested slowly and that will eliminate the dramatic highs and lows caused by sugar. You should try to include as many complex carbohydrates in your diet as you can. This week, focus on replacing sugary foods with complex carbohydrates like fresh fruits and vegetables, cereals, and whole-grain breads.

Your Sugar Risk

Are you aware of the effect sugar is having on how you feel each day? Or the effect it has on how you'll feel in the future? Here's a brief quiz that will help you see your sugar consumption in a new light:

1. Do you have a family history of diabetes?
2. Do you eat irregular meals at irregular times?
3. Do you drink sweetened soft drinks daily?
4. Do you eat cereals with sugar coating twice a week or more?

5. Do you drink tea or coffee with sugar daily?

6. Do you eat cookies, candy, ice cream, chocolate, cake, pies, doughnuts, etc., more than twice a week?

7. Do you ignore the sugar content of food listed on the labels when you shop?

8. If you go too long without eating, do you begin to feel tired, irritable, fatigued, or moody?

9. If you go too long without eating, do you get a headache?

10. If you go too long without eating, do you crave sweets?

11. Do you crave sweets at certain times of the day?

12. When you are under stress, do you crave sweets?

13. Do you have periods during the day when you feel tense and nervous, when you perspire and notice palpitations?

If you answered yes to more than three questions, your sugar consumption may be causing you undue fatigue. If you answered yes to six or more questions, your sugar consumption may be causing you to develop the symptoms of low blood sugar. If you answered yes to nine or more questions, and you have a family history of diabetes, you may be predisposing yourself to develop the disease.

Preparing for Week Two

Before you begin your sugar-free week, you'll need to do three things. My patients usually find it works best to begin each week of the Makeover on a weekend. If that works for you, begin preparing for Week Two at the end of your caffeine-free week.

1. First, read this entire chapter, particularly the

material that follows, which will familiarize you with hidden sources of sugar and will suggest substitutes for it.

2. Shop for groceries. You'll probably have to stock up on sugar-free snacks, drinks, desserts, salad dressings, etc. This doesn't entail a major investment, but it must be done in advance. If you wake up on Saturday morning with nothing to eat but heavily sweetened breakfast food, you're getting off to a bad start, and it's crucial that you begin the week on a positive note.

3. You have read about the supplement chromium in this chapter, and should buy some at your local drugstore or health-food store. Chromium is going to help keep your blood sugar on an even keel and control your sweet cravings.

What About "Natural" Sugars?

Many people have the mistaken notion that some sugars are good while others are bad. This simply isn't true. While there are over one hundred sweet substances that could be legitimately called sugar, sucrose, or table sugar, is the one we're most familiar with and the one most readily connected with the health hazards we've been discussing. But what about raw sugar? Or honey? Aren't they less "processed" and more "nutritional"? The answer is no. While some raw honey may have more vitamins than table sugar, most honey has been heat-processed and is devoid of nutrients. Raw sugar, brown sugar, turbinado sugar, maple syrup, or blackstrap molasses offer no real advantages over regular white sugar, and are not acceptable on the Medical Makeover. They cause all the blood-sugar and nutrition- and health-related problems we're trying to avoid.

Hidden Sugars: Learn to Read Labels

Even if you don't own a sugar bowl, half of your carbohydrate intake is probably in the form of sugar. Most of it is hidden in the foods you buy. No doubt you can name a number of products that contain sugar simply because they taste sweet. Canned fruits, sweet cereals, candy bars, and cookies obviously contain sugar. But if you rely solely on your taste buds to detect sugar in your food, you'll still be eating large quantities of it unawares. Sugar is used not only to sweeten food, but to preserve it, help prevent microbial deterioration, enhance yeast action, and aid in curing. The sugar in tomato products counteracts the acidity, the sugar in frozen desserts lowers the freezing point, and there's even sugar in iodized salt to stabilize the added iodide.

If you're going to cut sugar out of your diet, obviously you're going to have to become an informed consumer. Learn to read labels! Here are the most common sugar additives in your food:

- corn syrup
- sucrose
- fructose
- glucose
- lactose
- maltose
- molasses
- maple syrup
- sorghum

When you see sugar, or any of the forms of sugar additives listed above, on a label, don't buy that food. Once you begin to examine food labels, you'll notice many of them list one form of sugar as the second or third ingredient. Ingredients are shown in descending order of amounts used; so a product that counts sugar as its second ingredient probably has an enormous amount in it. Moreover, sometimes you'll notice that there are two or three forms of sugar listed. Though they may be near the bottom of the list of ingredients, thus lulling you into thinking that there's not much sugar in the product, if you added them up, sugar might be the main ingredient!

Don't depend on common sense when shopping for sugar-free foods. Many foods that you'd never guess have sugar in them, do. Soups, spaghetti sauces, ketchups, mayonnaises, cranberry sauces, and peanut butter are all examples of items that contain sugar. Remember that you don't have to eliminate all these items from your diet. It's possible, for example, to buy peanut butter without sugar: You can get it at a health food store. There are also one or two popular national brands that don't have sugar in them. The same goes for spaghetti sauces. You can find brands that don't contain sugar, but you have to search for them.

The following table will help you realize the extent to which hidden sugars contribute to your overall sugar intake.

REFINED SWEETENERS IN FOODS AND BEVERAGES

	Serving Size	Table Sugar Equivalent (tsps.)	Sugar Calories (% of total calories)
Sweeteners			
Pancake Syrup			
Karo Pancake & Waffle Syrup	1 tbs.	3.8	100
Golden Griddle	1 tbs.	3.3	100
Honey	1 tsp.	1.4	100
Table Sugar	1 tsp.	1	100
Molasses, light	1 tsp.	0.8	100

	Serving Size	Table Sugar Equivalent (tsps.)	Sugar Calories (% of total calories)
Soda Pop			
Patio Orange Soda	12 oz.	11.8	100
Shasta Orange Soda	12 oz.	11.8	100
Mountain Dew	12 oz.	11	100
On Tap Root Beer	12 oz.	10.3	100
Pepsi-Cola	12 oz.	10	100
Shasta Cola	12 oz.	9.8	100
Coca-Cola	12 oz.	9.3	100
Teem	12 oz.	9.3	100
Sprite	12 oz.	9	100
Canada Dry Tonic Water	12 oz.	8.4	97.7
Canada Dry Ginger Ale	12 oz.	8	94.8
Shasta Ginger Ale	12 oz.	8	100
Other Beverages			
Shasta Iced Tea	12 oz.	8.3	100
Ssips, Orange	8.45 oz.	7.3	89
PDQ Eggnog Flavor	2–3 tbs.	6.8	96
Hawaiian Punch	8 oz.	6.5	100
Carnation Chocolate Slender, canned	1 can	6.3	45
Kool-Aid, you add sugar	8 oz.	6.3	100
Country Time Lemonade Flavor, frozen concentrate	8 oz.	6	100
Kool-Aid, sugar already added	8 oz.	5.5–6	100
Capri Sun (all flavors)	1 bag	5.1–5.9	90
Country Time Lemonade Flavor, Ready to Drink	8 oz.	5.8	100
Nestlé Hot Cocoa Mix	1 oz.	5.8	84
Country Time Lemonade Flavor, Drink Mix	8 oz.	5.5	97.7
Hi-C, Grape	6 oz.	5.5	88

	Serving Size	Table Sugar Equivalent (tsps.)	Sugar Calories (% of total calories)
Nestlé Hot Cocoa Mix, with Marshmallows	1 oz.	5.5	80
Nestlé Strawberry Quik	2 tsp.	5.5	98
Carnation Strawberry Slender, canned	1 can	5.3*	38
Carnation Vanilla Slender, canned	1 can	5.3*	38
Cranberry Juice Cocktail	6 oz.	4.8	73
Nestlé Chocolate Quik	2 tsp.	4.5	80
Nestea Iced Tea Mix, Sugar & Lemon	6 oz.	4.3	97.1
Ovaltine Malt Flavor	4–5 tsp.	4.3	77
Carnation Milk Chocolate Hot Cocoa Mix	1 packet	4*	57
Ovaltine Chocolate Flavor	4–5 tsp.	4	82
PDQ Artificial Strawberry Flavor	3–4 tsp.	3.8	100
PDQ Chocolate Flavor	3–4 tsp.	3.8	91
Tang	4 oz.	3.8	100
Carnation Eggnog Instant Breakfast	1 packet	3.5*	43
Gatorade	8 oz.	3.5	100
Carnation Chocolate Instant Breakfast	1 packet	3*	37
Nestea Light	6 oz.	2.8	100
Carnation Instant Chocolate Malted Milk Cocoa Mix	3 tsp.	2.8*	52
Carnation Vanilla Instant Break.	1 packet	2.3*	28
Carnation Chocolate Slender, Instant	1 packet	2.3*	33
Carnation Vanilla Slender, Instant	1 packet	1.8*	25

*Sweetener figures include sucrose only.

	Serving Size	Table Sugar Equivalent (tsps.)	Sugar Calories (% of total calories)
Candy			
Jelly Beans	10 pieces	6.6	100
Marshmallows	0.9 oz.	4.8	100
M&M's			
Plain	1.7 oz.	6.8	46
Peanut	1.7 oz.	5.5	37
Candy Bars**			
Milky Way	2.1 oz.	9	21
Snickers	2.0 oz.	7.3	42
Mars bar	1.7 oz.	6.3	28
Royals	1.5 oz.	6.3	47
$100,000 bar	1.5 oz.	5.3	42
Reese's Peanut Butter Cups	1.6 oz.	5.3	31
Nestlé's Choco-Lite	1 oz.	4	43
Nestlé's Milk Chocolate	1 oz.	4	43
Hershey's Milk Chocolate	1 oz.	3.8	38
Hershey's Milk Chocolate, Almonds	1 oz.	3.5	35
Krackel	1 oz.	3.5	37
Nestlé's Crunch	1 oz.	3.5	37
Nestlé's Milk Chocolate, Almonds	1 oz.	3.5	37
Twix Caramel	0.9 oz.	3.3	40
Mr. Goodbar	1 oz.	3	31
Twix Peanut Butter	0.9 oz.	2.5	31
Summit Cookie Bars	0.7 oz.	2	28

**Roughly 10% of the sugar in chocolate bars is milk sugar (lactose).

Carnation Slender Bars*			
Chocolate Chip	2 bars	4.8	28
Chocolate	2 bars	4.3	25

*Sweetener figures include sucrose only.

	Serving Size	Table Sugar Equivalent (tsps.)	Sugar Calories (% of total calories)
Chocolate Peanut Butter	2 bars	4.3	25
Vanilla	2 bars	4.3	25
Lemon Yogurt	2 bars	4	24
Raspberry Yogurt	2 bars	4	24
Strawberry Yogurt	2 bars	4	24
Hard Candy			
Life Saver Lollipop	1 pop	2.8	100
Life Saver	1 piece	0.6	100
Life Saver Sours	1 piece	0.6	100
Life Saver Mint	1 piece	0.5	100
Gum			
Bubble Yum Bubble Gum	1 piece	1.8	100
Hubba Bubba	1 piece	1.5	100
Replay	1 piece	1.1	98.9
Fruit Stripe	1 piece	0.6	100
Wrigley, all stick varieties	1 piece	0.6	92
Beech-Nut	1 piece	0.6	98
Cough Drops			
Beech-Nut Cough Drops	1 piece	0.6	100
Pine Bros. Cough Drops	1 piece	0.6	98
Baked Goods			
Homemade Baked Goods			
Apple Pie à la Mode	2 oz.	3.5	24
Sponge Cake	1 oz.	3	48
Angel Food Cake	1 oz.	2	39
Pound Cake	1 oz.	1.8	20
Brownies with Nuts	0.7 oz.	1.6	27
Blueberry Muffins	1.4 oz.	0.8	12
Keebler Cookies			
Old Fashioned Oatmeal	2 pieces	2.5	25

	Serving Size	Table Sugar Equivalent (tsps.)	Sugar Calories (% of total calories)
Pitter Patter	2 pieces	2.5	22
Rich 'n Chips	2 pieces	2.5	25
Vanilla Wafers	7 pieces	2.3	28
Coconut Chocolate Drop	2 pieces	2	19
Elfwich	2 pieces	2	29
CC Biggs Chocolate Chip	2 pieces	1.8	25
Fudge Covered Graham Crackers	2 pieces	1.8	35
Fudge Stripes	2 pieces	1.8	25
Pecan Sandies	2 pieces	1.5	14
Double Nutty Peanut Butter	2 pieces	1.3	15
Kellogg's Pop-Tarts			
Frosted Chocolate Vanilla	1 tart	4.8	35
Frosted Brown Sugar & Cinnamon	1 tart	3.5	27
Blueberry or Cherry Filled	1 tart	3.3	25
Twinkies	1 pkg.	8.4	47
Sara Lee Chocolate Cake	1.7 oz.	4.2	37
Graham Crackers	2 pieces	0.9	25
Dairy Products			
Low-Fat Yogurt, fruit	1 cup	7.5	52
Frozen Yogurt, whole milk	4 oz.	6.1	62
Yogurt, flavored	1 cup	4.1	34
Vanilla Ice Milk	½ cup	3.4	48
Dannon Frozen Yogurt, Fruit	½ cup	3.3	50

	Serving Size	Table Sugar Equivalent (tsps.)	Sugar Calories (% of total calories)
Vanilla Ice Cream	½ cup	3.2	37
Dannon Frozen Yogurt, Vanilla	½ cup	2.8	50
Chocolate Milk, 2% fat	1 cup	2.7	24

Other Desserts and Sweet Snacks

Popsicle	1	4.5	100
Hunt's Snack Pack, Vanilla	1 can	4.4	37
Chocolate Pudding, homemade	½ cup	3.9	39
Canned Pears, heavy syrup	½ cup	3.6	59
Canned Pineapple, heavy syrup	½ cup	3	54
Orange Sherbet	½ cup	2.8	33

Breakfast Cereals***
General Mills

Boo Berry	1 oz.	3.3	47
Count Chocula	1 oz.	3.3	47
Franken Berry	1 oz.	3.3	47
Chocolate Crazy Cow	1 oz.	3	44
Pac-Man	1 oz.	3	44
Strawberry Shortcake	1 oz.	3	44
Trix	1 oz.	3	44
Cocoa Puffs	1 oz.	2.8	40
Lucky Charms	1 oz.	2.8	40
Cheerios, Honey Nut	1 oz.	2.5	36
Donutz, Chocolate Flavor	1 oz.	2.5	33
Donutz, Powdered	1 oz.	2.5	33
Golden Grahams	1 oz.	2.5	36

****Figures for cereals include naturally occurring sugar in raisins and other dried fruits.*

	Serving Size	Table Sugar Equivalent (tsps.)	Sugar Calories (% of total calories)
Buc Wheats	1 oz.	2.3	33
Nature Valley Granola, Fruit & Nut	1 oz.	2	25
Nature Valley Granola, Cinnamon & Raisin	1 oz.	1.8	22
Body Buddies, Brown Sugar & Honey	1 oz.	1.5	22
Body Buddies, Fruit Flavor	1 oz.	1.5	22
Kaboom	1 oz.	1.5	22
Nature Valley Granola, Coconut & Honey	1 oz.	1.5	16
Nature Valley Granola, Toasted Oat	1 oz.	1.5	18
Country Corn Flakes	1 oz.	0.8	11
Total	1 oz.	0.8	11
Total, Corn	1 oz.	0.8	11
Wheaties	1 oz.	0.8	11
Kix	1 oz.	0.5	7
Cheerios	1 oz.	0.3	4
Kellogg's			
Honey Smacks	1 oz.	4	58
Apple Jacks	1 oz.	3.5	51
Froot Loops	1 oz.	3.3	47
Cocoa Krispies	1 oz.	3	44
Sugar Corn Pops	1 oz.	3	44
Frosted Flakes, Sugar	1 oz.	2.8	40
Frosted Flakes, Banana	1 oz.	2.5	36
Frosted Krispies	1 oz.	2.5	36
Marshmallow Krispies	1 oz.	2.5	29
Raisins, Rice & Rye	1 oz.	2.5	29
Strawberry Krispies	1 oz.	2.5	36
Corn Flakes, Honey & Nut	1 oz.	2.3	33
Cracklin' Oat Bran	1 oz.	2	27

	Serving Size	Table Sugar Equivalent (tsps.)	Sugar Calories (% of total calories)
Nutri-Grain, Wheat & Raisins	1 oz.	2	23
Bran Buds	1 oz.	1.8	40
Frosted Mini-Wheats, Sugar-Frosted	1 oz.	1.8	25
Frosted Mini-Wheats, Apple-Flavored	1 oz.	1.8	25
Most	1 oz.	1.5	24
All-Bran	1 oz.	1.3	29
40% Bran Flakes	1 oz.	1.3	22
Crispix	1 oz.	0.8	11
Product 19	1 oz.	0.8	11
Rice Krispies	1 oz.	0.8	11
Special K	1 oz.	0.8	11
Corn Flakes	1 oz.	0.5	7
Nutri-Grain, Corn	1 oz.	0.5	7
Nutri-Grain, Wheat	1 oz.	0.5	7
Post			
Super Sugar Crisp	1 oz.	3.5	51
Honeycomb	1 oz.	2.8	40
Raisin Bran	1 oz.	2.3	40
Fruit & Fibre	1 oz.	1.8	31
Raisin Grape Nuts	1 oz.	1.5	24
40% Bran Flakes	1 oz.	1.3	22
Grape Nut Flakes	1 oz.	1.3	20
Grape Nuts	1 oz.	0.8	12
Ralston Purina			
Cookie Crisp, Choc. Chip Flavor	1 oz.	3.3	47
Cookie Crisp, Vanilla Wafer	1 oz.	3.3	47
Donkey Kong Junior	1 oz.	3.3	47
Cookie Crisp, Oatmeal Flavor	1 oz.	3	40

	Serving Size	Table Sugar Equivalent (tsps.)	Sugar Calories (% of total calories)
Sugar Frosted Flakes	1 oz.	2.8	40
Raisin Bran	1 oz.	2.3	36
Bran Chex	1 oz.	1.3	18
Crispy Rice	1 oz.	0.8	11
Corn Chex	1 oz.	0.5	7
Corn Flakes	1 oz.	0.5	7
Rice Chex	1 oz.	0.5	7
Wheat Chex	1 oz.	0.5	7
Quaker Oats			
Cap'n Crunch's Crunchberries	1 oz.	3.3	43
Cap'n Crunch	1 oz.	3	44
King Vitaman	1 oz.	3	44
Quisp	1 oz.	3	44
Cap'n Crunch's Peanut Butter	1 oz.	2.5	31
100% Natural, Raisins & Dates	1 oz.	2.3	28
100% Natural, Apples & Cinnamon	1 oz.	2	23
Life, Cinnamon	1 oz.	1.5	22
100% Natural	1 oz.	1.5	17
Life	1 oz.	1.3	18
Shredded Wheat	1.3 oz.	0.3	3
Puffed Rice	0.5 oz.	0	0
Puffed Wheat	0.5 oz.	0	0
Miscellaneous			
Cranberry Sauce	1 tbs.	1.5	96
Skippy Peanut Butter	2 tbs.	1.3	11
Ketchup	1 tbs.	0.6	63

Sweetener amounts are manufacturers' approximations or are CSPI (Center for Science in the Public Interest) estimates based on data supplied by manufacturers.

The Cold-Turkey Approach

I think it's important to avoid sugar completely, at least for the duration of the Medical Makeover. By keeping your system clear of sugar, it will be easier to regain a normal metabolism. You'll eliminate the highs and lows that you experience when you eat sugar.

There's a psychological aspect to the cold-turkey approach: As with giving up caffeine, if you have just a little bit, it makes it difficult to justify complete abstention. Perhaps you have just a teaspoon of sugar on some cereal and you don't think it affects you very much. That experience tempts you to have just a bit more sugar on another occasion. Before you know it, you're right back where you started. It's much easier to make an iron-clad rule for yourself in the beginning and, at least during the Makeover, stick with it. That way you're eliminating as many decisions as possible, and making decisions when you're tired or stressed or fatigued is how willpower becomes eroded.

There's another reason to give up sugar completely. After a period of time without it, you'll find that the strength of your sweet tooth diminishes. Many things that you enjoyed in the past will begin to taste overly sweet to you.

Bill F., an advertising space salesman for a leading magazine, came to see me because he was having persistent morning headaches. When I discussed his diet with him, I discovered he had a powerful sweet tooth. He would have a bowl of ice cream in the evening after work, and then an hour later he would want another. On some nights he would have four or five bowls of ice cream. He never made the connection between his early-morning headaches and his ice cream binges, but one always followed the other. He weighed 213 pounds on his first visit, and, though disheartened by his weight, he was more concerned about the headaches. When I told him he had to give up sugar, he was resistant. Ice cream gave him so much pleasure that he didn't think he could bear to give it up. Besides, he couldn't believe that the sugar had anything to do with his headaches. I urged him to go sugar-free for just two weeks. He was willing to try it for just that long and no longer.

When Bill's two sugar-free weeks were over, he was pleased to report that his sweet tooth had virtually disappeared. The combination of the chromium and his newly stabilized metabolism had made it much easier to avoid sugar, even in tempting situations. And his headaches were gone too. He has been off sugar now for nearly a year. He told me that he was recently served a piece of wedding cake at a reception and after a few bites couldn't eat any more. It seemed sickeningly sweet.

You'll discover that if you give up sugar completely for a period of time, your sense of taste will be sharpened and you'll lose your addiction to sugar. You'll taste the real flavor of things and won't yearn for the sweetness that typically masks the flavor of food.

What About Sugar Substitutes?

Just as it's important to go cold turkey when you give up sugar, I think that using sugar substitutes is a half measure. For one thing, it foils your effort to reeducate your taste buds; sugar substitutes simply encourage you to continue to crave that sweet taste. Moreover, if you're continually eating sweet things, it's too easy to be tempted to have a sugar-sweetened cola if you can't get an artificially sweetened one. Most people use an artificial sweetener because they think it helps keep their weight down. You may be lulled into believing that you're getting something for nothing, but no study has ever shown that the use of artificial sweeteners has been of any use whatsoever either in weight control or the control of diabetes. Finally, despite FDA approval, there is lingering evidence that artificial sweeteners can cause health problems.

Here's the latest information on the two most popular artificial sweeteners:

Aspartame, which was approved for use in soft drinks in 1983, has nearly the same number of calories by weight as sugar but is two hundred times sweeter. This means that the amount needed to sweeten something is so tiny as to be virtually noncaloric. Aspartame is very popular because its taste is very close to that of natural sugar. However, there have been reports that some people suffer from severe headaches, depression, or seizures after consuming aspartame. In addition, some tests have shown that aspartame causes brain tumors in rats and could be cancer-causing to humans. There is also some evidence that the amount of aspartame that an adult might safely consume could cause brain damage in a child or in the fetus of a pregnant woman. These studies are still controversial in that there is some conflicting evidence.

Saccharin is an artificial sweetener that has been around for a long time. It is probably the one you are most familiar with. Saccharin is three hundred times sweeter than sugar, but it does have a bitter aftertaste. Worse than the bitter aftertaste is the link between saccharin and bladder cancer in laboratory rats. Though that study has been discounted by saccharin supporters, the results demonstrated that 3 percent of rats fed a diet of 5 percent saccharin from birth developed bladder cancers and, worse, 14 percent of their offspring fed the same diet also developed cancers. Applied to humans, this means that three people out of one hundred would develop bladder cancer if they drank just a single can of diet soda each day for a lifetime. (And very few people who drink diet soda limit themselves to one a day!)

In 1977 when studies revealed this problem and there was talk of banning saccharin, it was the only artificial sweetener around. Because of public devotion to saccharin, the ban on it was delayed for eighteen months so further studies could be done. This ban has been delayed three times for eighteen-month periods. As of this writing the latest extension is about to expire, and it looks as if yet another one will be granted. Some studies demonstrate that saccharin is safe, but others support the claim that it's a carcinogen with no known safe level for consumption.

I think that the data on artificial sweeteners indicate consumers should be cautious. We can't be absolutely positive that these sweeteners are safe. Moreover, as I've said, they encourage you to yearn for the sweet taste that ties you to sugar. Finally, there's some evidence that artificial sweeteners foil the very purpose we use them for: to keep weight down by cutting down on calories. There's some evidence that the use of saccharin stimulates the appetite and interferes with the regulation of blood sugar. This puts a stress on the body and, in addition to affecting physical health, can contribute to the emotional lows that cause you to overeat. Obviously, for our purposes, the use of artificial sweeteners is counterproductive.

Tips for Success

It's not difficult to give up sugar, but it takes more planning than giving up caffeine because sugar is hiding everywhere and sometimes in the most unlikely places. You must plan ahead. You have to shop with care before you even begin the week, and you have to anticipate your meals and snacks. You can't prepare a salad only to realize there's only Russian dressing in the house and it's loaded with sugar. Here are some tips—some my own and others gleaned from my patients—that will help you through the week and the rest of your sugar-free Medical Makeover:

• The best BREAKFAST FOODS are cereals like oatmeal, Wheatena, or plain shredded wheat. They'll fill you up and have no added sugar. Fresh fruit will give some sweetness and texture. One of my patients who thought she couldn't live without sweet breakfast cereal found that adding some raisins to it gave her all the sweetness she wanted.

• YOGURT makes a good breakfast if you have with it some whole-wheat toast or perhaps a bran muffin for fiber. But don't buy the kind with fruit. Buy low-fat plain yogurt and add fresh fruit yourself. A combination of orange and banana pieces, or grapes and melon balls, is especially nice. I always add a sprinkling of oat bran (available in health food stores) to yogurt for fiber, texture, and vitamins.

• PLAN YOUR LUNCH. Don't just run to the deli unless you know in advance what sugar-free foods they have. One of my patients, Linda G., who works for a small advertising agency, fell into this trap. She told me, "I thought I was doing something healthy when I had a ham or tuna sandwich at the deli. I'd get some cole slaw to go with it and a diet soda. But I often noticed that after lunch I'd start to sweat. Now I realize that I was eating large amounts of sugar and, like many people who are having too much sugar, that was what was responsible for the sweats. The ham, the tuna, the roll, the cole slaw— they were all made with sugar. And to top if off, I'd often have a sweet in the afternoon. Now I'll bring a piece of chicken from home and a bit of low-fat cheese and a homemade salad. It takes a little longer, but I do it the night before and I've gotten used to it."

• A popular standby for my patients who don't have

time to fix lunch in advance is cans of TUNA PACKED IN WATER. With some plain salad, and toast or crackers and fruit, plain tuna can make a satisfying lunch.

• If you like to bake, you can cut down on a lot of sugar by MAKING THINGS FROM SCRATCH. I always used to think that if you were going to eat a muffin or some bread, it didn't really make much difference whether you made it or bought it. That was until I learned what is contained in most commercially baked items. Corn syrup is often used as a sweetener in commercially baked products. Corn syrup is cheap, plentiful, and easy to use, but the only problem is it's not as sweet as table sugar. So large amounts of corn syrup are added to get the desired sweetness. When you eat these corn-syrup-sweetened items, you're getting even more "sugar" than if you had made them yourself using a standard recipe. And by the way, most standard recipes call for more sugar than necessary. You can usually cut the recommended amount by one third or even more.

• BAN DIET SODAS from your house. Instead, stock up on mineral water or seltzer water. Three or four parts of seltzer water to one part fruit juice makes a refreshing drink. Or drink the water plain with a slice of lemon, lime, or orange. I keep plain seltzer water in my office and drink it frequently during the day. I add just a squeeze of lemon juice from one of those plastic lemons.

• If you can't find commercial sugar-free products, try to MAKE YOUR OWN without sugar. If you use a lot of mayonnaise and can't find a sugar-free kind, make your own. It's not difficult to do, and you can make it in a blender if you have one. You can also make salad dressings by mixing yogurt, buttermilk, garlic, and herbs in the blender.

• FRESH FRUITS are best, but you can buy canned fruit packed in its own juices. In the winter, this fruit over homemade, sugar-free biscuits with a yogurt topping makes a nice shortcake.

• CHECK PICKLE LABELS. Many pickles, though not all, contain sugar. As I rarely eat them, I wasn't aware of this fact, but a patient said he had been eating lots of pickles, thinking that they couldn't possibly have sugar in them—until he checked the label!

• UNBUTTERED POPCORN makes a good substitute for a sweet snack in the evening, or any time of day, for that matter. There are even hot-air machines available that allow you to make it at home without any oil.

Analyze Your Triggers

SOCIAL SITUATIONS can be your downfall if you're not prepared. It can be tough to be the only one at a dinner party not eating the specially prepared dessert. Hostesses have been known to become overbearing in such situations. One of my patients told me that he simply tells people he's "prediabetic." In fact, he does have a family history of the disease, and what "prediabetic" means is that if he doesn't watch his sugar intake, he's likely to develop diabetes. But his wife, who has no family history of diabetes, tells people that she's prediabetic, too, when she doesn't want to eat sweets. Somehow an actual "diagnosis" sounds more serious than just that you're cutting out sugar. One patient, a clinical psychologist, told me that one time when she was visiting her mother, she had been pressured into eating cookies her mother had prepared for her even though she had informed her mother she couldn't have sugar. She told me that night she had a hard time sleeping, and she's convinced that it was because of the sugar—the only sugar she had had in weeks. The next time she will tell her mother that she can't eat a thing right now but that she would love to take the cookies home to eat later. That way she can avoid hurting her mother's feelings by discarding the cookies when she reaches home.

One of my patients told me that the hardest time for her to avoid sweets was in a restaurant when everyone was ORDERING DESSERT. She has come up with an excellent delaying tactic. When the waiter takes the dessert order, she says, "I'll just have some tea for now and see if I feel like something later." (She always carries herbal tea bags with her in case the restaurant has none.) This assertive statement deflects the comments from fellow diners who used to encourage her to order dessert too. And of course by the time she has finished the tea, everyone else has finished dessert and forgotten she never ordered one.

IF YOU MUST, ABSOLUTELY MUST, HAVE SOMETHING SWEET—and I hope you can at least get through a few sugar-free weeks before you give in to the irresistible urge—then be sure to have it after a meal and not on an empty stomach. Sugar eaten after a meal takes longer to enter your bloodstream and begin the high/low effect that can wreak havoc with your metabolism.

Enlist Helpers

As in all the weeks of the Medical Makeover, you're going to need the SUPPORT OF YOUR FAMILY AND FRIENDS. Giving up sugar is so important that you should try to convert your family at the same time. If you have children or teenagers, you may have a challenge on your hands, but in fact they can probably use a reduction in sugar even more than you. Among young people excess sugar consumption has been linked to everything from hyperactivity to malnutrition. Make the sugar-free week a challenge for them and explain how important it is for you. Tell them it won't last forever—at the end of the Makeover you may re-introduce a certain amount of sugar into your and their diets. But try not to have sweet snacks around the house, as it only makes it more difficult for you, and it certainly doesn't help your children in the long or the short run.

Dealing with Relapse

As I said in the chapter on caffeine, it's important not to castigate yourself too severely if you break down and have a sweet. Don't decide you'll never succeed with the Makeover, that you are a failure, that everything you do ends in failure, so you might as well have another piece of chocolate. See your slip for what it is: a small step backward, nothing more. Say to yourself, "So, OK, I did it, but it's not the end of the world, and now I'll go right back to my plan of avoiding sweets. I can do it." And you will.

Week Three: The New Nutrition

- Do you skip breakfast, have a light lunch and a full dinner?
- Do you sometimes have such a busy day that you eat dinner after 9:00 P.M.?
- Do you believe that you've never been able to stick with a diet because of lack of willpower?

If you're like many of my patients, you're living with a few myths and misconceptions about nutrition that are keeping you from enjoying optimum health. Your nutrition isn't really *bad*, but a change—a fine tuning—of your approach to eating could improve every aspect of your life from daily energy and enthusiasm to ultimate life span.

Now that you've eliminated two unhealthy habits— caffeine and sugar—you're ready to take *positive* measures to improve your health. Your metabolism is already better stabilized: You've probably discovered that any energy slumps or periods of fatigue that you used to suffer during the day are gone. Because you are no longer experiencing the high and low levels of blood sugar caused by caffeine and sweets, you're much more able to control what and when you eat.

This week is not difficult—it's not like any other "diet" that you might have tried and failed with. It's a simple, unique approach to good nutrition. Still, you may have to make some changes in your life-style because eating is one of our most sociable and pleasant activities. You may have some bad habits to break that involve other people— the family and friends you eat with. On the other hand, many of my patients find that a lot of their bad eating habits are solitary—the skipped breakfast, the high-calorie snacking, the late, large dinner. You, too, may find that changing your eating habits isn't as hard as it could be because your unhealthy eating patterns can be changed to healthy ones in very pleasurable ways.

This Week's Goal

By the end of this week you are going to be better nourished. You are already eating regular meals at fairly regular times. You have some idea of good nutrition, but there are weak spots where you indulge yourself for any number of reasons. This week you're going to try to eliminate those weak spots.

While the Medical Makeover may cause you to lose weight, that's not its primary goal. I tell my patients that if they begin the nutrition improvement week thinking only of weight control, they're likely to defeat themselves. So, at least for now, forget about weight and think about positive nutrition.

For many people this week is more of a shift than a complete change. It may have seemed impossible to give up caffeine and sugar, but you did it. That was a dramatic change. Improving your nutrition is not a dramatic change, but it's more complex. You have to pay more attention, especially in the beginning. Once you've developed your own healthy eating plan, and gotten used to it, it will be easy to stick with it.

Your taste buds will have more of a yearning for, say, a chef's salad with lots of fresh vegetables than for a fast-food double burger which will begin to seem too greasy and fatty and salty to you.

Once again, read this chapter all the way through. You may have to do some food shopping, and you must do it in advance. You don't want to wake up on Sunday or Monday morning ready to have a good breakfast only to find that there's nothing in the house to eat but some leftover Chinese takeout food and a half-bottle of ketch-up. The second half of this chapter has lots of practical tips on how to achieve a healthy diet, and it might be useful to jot down a shopping list. That way, you won't have to keep all the items you might want to buy in your head.

Evaluating Your Nutrition

Here's a quick quiz that will help you to recognize the weak spots in your diet:

1. Do you eat regular meals at regular times?
2. Do you eat breakfast?
3. Do you eat fresh fruits and vegetables daily?
4. Do you eat whole grains and fiber daily?
5. Do you read food package labels to minimize your intake of fats, sugars, and preservatives?
6. Do you avoid white-flour products?
7. Do you avoid fried food, including fast foods?
8. Do you avoid fats such as butter, margarine, cheese, mayonnaise, oils, etc?
9. Do you eat fewer than three eggs per week?
10. Do you avoid red meat?

11. Do you avoid using table salt?
12. Do you avoid sugar and sweetened foods like cookies and candy as well as artificial sweeteners suc as those found in diet sodas?
13. Do you drink no more than one cup of coffee a day?

If you answered no to more than three questions, your eating habits may be predisposing you to daily fatigue as well as possible heart disease and cancer in the future.

Death by the Forkful:
The Changing American Diet

Your grandfather may have been healthier than you are even though he lived in an era whose sanitation was primitive by today's standards, with no antibiotics or immunizations and with unsophisticated medical techniques. If he could have enjoyed the benefits of modern medicine back then, he would probably have lived longer than you will. Why? Because of better nutrition. He ate less meat, far less sugar, virtually no processed foods, and drank less alcohol than you do. He also ate more grain products, more fresh fruit and vegetables.

Today, largely because of their diets, over 50 percent of all Americans are at risk for heart disease, diabetes, hypertension, and cancer. In 1977, George McGovern headed a congressional committee that investigated the American diet. The McGovern committee studied the relationship between this diet and the nation's major killers—heart disease, cancers of the colon and breast, stroke, high blood pressure, obesity, diabetes, arteriosclerosis, and cirrhosis of the liver. They estimated that if Americans modified their rich diets, there would be an 80 percent drop in the number of obese people, a 25 percent drop in deaths from heart disease, a 50 percent drop in deaths from diabetes, and a 1 percent annual increase in longevity.

Most people are well aware of at least some of the problems with the average American diet. They know they should be eating less fat and red meat, more fish, poultry, fresh vegetables, and fruits. Every week, it seems, a new study confirms the havoc we are wreaking with our health by eating the way we do. Our diet is far too rich in meats, dairy products, alcohol, and processed foods that are laden with fats, cholesterol, sugar, salt, and calories.

Even though public consciousness has been raised to some degree about improved nutrition, it's interesting to remember that as recently as five years ago, some of the principles we accept as givens were controversial. Believe it or not, as late as 1980 *The New York Times* featured a front-page article with the headline "PANEL REPORTS HEALTHY AMERICANS NEED NOT CUT INTAKE OF CHOLESTEROL." The article stated that the Food and Nutrition Board of the National Research Council said it had found "no clearcut evidence that reducing blood levels of cholesterol by dietary changes could prevent coronary heart disease. It said further that the fat and cholesterol modifications recommended by other groups had not been shown to be entirely free of risk."

In 1984 another panel convened by the National Institutes of Health made the front page of *The New York Times*. It said that the "average cholesterol levels among Americans were too high [levels that have been considered "normal" by many physicians] and contributed to the fact that half the population died of heart disease." The panel recommended dietary changes to lower cholesterol, completely reversing their position of four years earlier! I believe this rapid change indicates that we are just at the beginning of major nutritional breakthroughs that will dramatically alter the way we view our diets. This emerging awareness can be referred to as the "New Nutrition."

How the New Nutrition Can Change Your Life

Unfortunately, it's been my experience over the years that the threat of future disease isn't enough to get my patients to change the way they eat. Even though improving their diet would probably be the single most effective step they could take toward avoiding chronic disease. Knowing, for example, that calorie and fat restriction have proven to have the most important influence on the reduction of cancer in humans probably won't encourage them to cut down on fats, even if they have a family history of cancer. My patients, however, are willing to change their eating habits because they are already feeling the effects of a poor diet. They're tired and irritable. They can't concentrate. They're vulnerable to colds and infections. They feel run down. They're willing at least to take a chance that better nutrition will help them.

What I discovered is that the diet that will help my patients avoid chronic disease in the future is the same diet that makes them feel better right away. This was a revelation to me as well as to them. I recommended that they follow nutritional guidelines similar to those proposed by the Surgeon General, the National Cancer Institute, and the American Heart Association. These guidelines, which were established to help people avoid the major causes of death and disease in America, can also help you feel more vital, calm, and energetic immediately. You don't have to wait for thirty years to see if the diet works; you'll be able to see its effects in a few days. I know it sounds dramatic but it's true. (Of course, this assumes that you've already given up caffeine and sugar. Otherwise, your blood sugar will still experience peaks and valleys that will affect the way you feel, and good nutrition can't entirely mitigate it.)

In addition to helping you avoid future disease and making you feel better right now, the New Nutrition can help your body withstand everyday stress. In other words, it can be a sort of insurance policy that will protect you against the tension and pressure that are inevitably assaulting your body. We have seen how coping with stress can take its toll. The New Nutrition gives your body the resilience it needs to withstand that stress; and when your body copes effectively with stress, at the same time it is protecting itself from future disease.

Why This Is Not a "Diet"

When I first began to help my patients improve their nutrition, I would give them a printed diet and suggest that they follow it. It wasn't a complicated diet. It gave recommended foods and amounts for each meal, and made suggestions about which foods to avoid and which to emphasize. The results were mixed at best. Some people followed the diet, but most did not. Or they would try to follow it for a few days or a week, and then they would stop. And when they failed to continue with the diet, they became discouraged, and some even told me that they were afraid to come in to see me because they had given up on the diet. Obviously, a traditional diet wasn't helping my patients improve their nutrition.

I've since come to believe that the typical "diet," which is usually a weight-reduction diet, is counterproductive. Not only is it counterproductive psychologically, it's counterproductive physically.

From a psychological standpoint, it's very discouraging to fail at something. When we try to perform a task and meet with failure, we can't help but establish an attitude, even subconsciously, that derides our original goal. With dieting, the basic approach is usually negative: Don't eat this, don't eat that, don't eat so much, don't eat so often. The dieter spends most of his or her time avoiding food. When he breaks down and goes off the diet, which is inevitable, he feels he has failed. He has no willpower, no strength of purpose. This sense of failure inspires the "what-the-hell" attitude. "I ate that doughnut this morning so, what the hell, I'll have a piece of cake at lunch." The diet is seen as an all-or-nothing proposition. There's success or failure and no middle ground. Once the what-the-hell attitude develops, it signals the beginning of the end of the diet, and there's almost a childish pleasure in flouting the rules even though the only one to suffer is the dieter.

The other psychological problem with diets is that most of them are supposed to be followed for a limited amount of time. They promise that if you change your eating habits for one or two or six weeks, you'll lose five or ten or thirty pounds and then you can go back to business as usual. Even the diets that claim that they will permanently improve your eating habits often propose menus or recipes that are difficult to follow. Somehow these diets never seem to work in the real world. They don't take into account business lunches, limited time for breakfast, business entertaining, a family who is not dieting with you, or what you can serve for dessert when you're on a diet and your guests are not.

The Biochemical Effects of Dieting

Dieting is not only psychologically trying, it's also physically debilitating and can actually cause you to gain, not lose, weight. Paul Ernsberger of Northwestern University recently published an article on what he calls the "yo-yo" syndrome—constantly trying and failing at weight-loss diets. He found that any sequence of diets not only sets a pattern that encourages weight gain, it also has severe health consequences.

If you diet constantly, and 42 percent of the readers of a national women's magazine said they did, you are constantly raising your weight baseline. Every time you restrict your calorie intake this forces your body to respond as if to starvation conditions. It reacts to lowered calories by conserving energy and lowering your metabolic pacemaker. It is prepared now to get by on less food. Of course, once you go off the diet and begin to eat more calories, your body reacts by gaining weight. It was prepared to function on fewer calories, so it stores the extra ones as fat. You're worse off than you were before the diet. Not only have you failed and become discouraged, you're fatter. This is a case where your metabolism—changed by dieting—works against your intentions, not with them.

Chronic dieters, and it seems there is no other kind, may commonly develop what's known as "dieter's hypertension." We have known for a long time that high blood pressure is common in people who are overweight, but it has been thought that this is a result of the extra weight. It turns out that the elevated pressure may in fact be a result of efforts to get rid of the weight.

Remember the antistress hormones epinephrine and norepinephrine? The body secretes norepinephrine in the face of stress, and it affects countless bodily functions as it prepares us for fight or flight. We saw that stress can be a loud noise or a threat from a mugger, but it can also be a drop in blood sugar. The body can become stressed when it doesn't function smoothly. So it is with dieting. Overeating, or increasing your daily caloric intake following a diet, can also be a stress on the body. When you overeat, your body prepares to get rid of the excess calories by going on a calorie-wasting binge. It has a system that actually "wastes" energy to dispose of a sudden onslaught of extra calories. But it takes norepinephrine to get this sytem going, and while the hormone is stimulating the energy-wasting system, it's also speeding up the heart and driving up the blood pressure.

This is probably why most diets encourage or allow

you to drink black coffee or diet soda. The caffeine stimulates the production of epinephrine and norepinephrine, and this helps you deal with the biochemical stress of dieting. Paradoxically, what you are actually doing is setting yourself up for a fall, for once you begin to reduce caffeine consumption—say, when the diet is over—you'll feel hungrier than before. And you'll probably eat more, quickly gaining back what you lost.

There have always been criticisms of diets and dieting from a health standpoint, but now the evidence seems to be overwhelming. However, not only are diets unhealthy, they fail at their basic goal: to help people lose weight permanently.

Weight Loss and the New Nutrition

As I've said, the New Nutrition is not geared specifically to weight loss; it's geared to health. I try to get my patients to think of weight loss as a side effect, particularly when they begin to change their eating habits. At the same time, many of them lose desired weight on the program. For one thing, if you give up sugar for any length of time, you almost have to lose weight because you're reducing your daily caloric intake. And when you adopt the principles of the New Nutrition, you'll find that they're not so different from the principles of a healthy weight-reducing diet. You'll be cutting down on fats and increasing fiber, increasing your fish and poultry intake. You'll also be lowering your red meat consumption and learning about how different foods affect your appetite in unexpected ways, and how certain foods affect your moods—in short, a whole battery of techniques that aid the dieter.

The fact is that many of my patients do want to lose weight. Very few of them are obese but many are eager to shed from five to fifteen pounds. They have found that the New Nutrition works, and it works better than any other method they've used to lose weight. Pat has lost a great deal of weight. She has gone from a size 16 to a size 7. She told me that she had always been chunky, that she had a tendency to gain weight ever since she was a child. Over a period of years—she is twenty-seven now—she had been on every conceivable diet. She did lose weight on some of them, but she never kept it off, and her biggest complaint is that the diets always made her feel hungry. She came to see me because she had been feeling tired and run down for a few months. She was getting colds often and felt depressed, and, worst of all from her point of view, she couldn't seem to stop eating. She didn't know if she was eating because she was depressed and tired, or if the eating and weight gain were making her depressed and tired.

When Pat first came to see me, I told her to forget about losing weight, at least for a few weeks, and just follow the principles of the New Nutrition as closely as she could. After she felt really healthy, then we would gear her diet to weight loss. But I think what was more important for her to hear was that her weight gain was not her fault. It didn't signal a character weakness. It was simply the result of eating the wrong foods. I told her that she would find that once she changed her eating habits, she would feel better, healthier. And she wouldn't be hungry. Within two months, Pat was a different person. She had already lost nearly fifteen pounds, slowly but steadily, and this was before we even modified her diet toward a weight-reducing plan. As Pat says today, "I hadn't realized how guilty I'd been feeling about gaining weight. I felt so depressed about it that it just made me want to eat more. It was really self-destructive. But when the focus became eating foods that were good for me and when there was no pressure to lose weight, I began to feel better right away. I felt that I was in control. This was something I could do. From the first day of the New Nutrition, I really acted like a thin person. Also from the first day, I felt that I looked wonderful."

Pat is an example of how a positive approach to nutrition can change the effectiveness of a weight-loss program. If you focus on the positive—eating healthy meals, taking care of your body, helping yourself to feel great—you change the dynamics of "dieting." The emphasis is on self-control, not self-denial. You're no longer depriving yourself. You're in charge. This is a much more important principle than it might seem at first glance.

Your Biochemical Boosters

By now you are taking *chromium* supplements on a daily basis to steady your blood-sugar fluctuations so you won't need a sweet pick-me-up when your blood sugar falls. You will recall that by having eliminated sugar, your body is not pumping out insulin, which increases your appetite.

By learning which foods rate high on the *glycemic index,* you should be avoiding those which act like sugar or glucose on the body, once again causing insulin levels to elevate. And make you hungry.

Now I'll add a new biochemical booster. I recommend taking *L-tryptophan* in doses of 500 milligrams. It's best taken on an empty stomach. This amino acid is converted to a brain neurotransmitter, serotonin, which appears to reduce carbohydrate cravings, the bane of anyone trying to lose weight. Although the point of this week is not to lose weight, it's often snacks between meals that throw our best intentions for good nutrition out the window.

Dr. Richard Wurtman of the Massachusetts Institute of Technology found that when the brain had a shortage of serotonin, it would develop a craving for carbohydrates.

He and his wife, Dr. Judith Wurtman, a nutritionist, studied obese individuals who craved carbohydrates between meals when serotonin levels were depressed. These individuals ate carbohydrate snacks, which started the insulin cascade, ultimately allowing tryptophan to enter the brain. In the brain the tryptophan was converted to serotonin, and the carbohydrate craving was temporarily satisfied.

Additionally, it appears that carbohydrate cravings are related to feeling depressed for no apparent reason. When the overweight patients in the Wurtmans' study were asked how they felt when they were craving carbohydrates, they said they were anxious, tense, unhappy. After eating a carbohydrate snack, they soon felt less tense, even relaxed. My patients report that taking tryptophan directly reduces or eliminates the desire for carbohydrate snacks. What tryptophan does is act directly on the brain to increase your serotonin level, which keeps your brain from telling you that it wants something to eat—*now*. Like a candy bar, or a cheese Danish.

Some of you may be aware that tryptophan induces sleep. To use it for that purpose, you need to take 1,500 milligrams before bedtime. Taken in the smaller dosage I recommend for the Makeover and spaced throughout the day, it won't make you sleepy.

Establishing New Eating Habits

In addition to the biochemical boosters, your eating habits also play a major role in stabilizing your metabolism. You may already be doing some of the things I'm going to suggest—growing up, you probably heard them from your grandmother—but I've found that a great many people don't take these eating habits seriously. Maybe you don't either. But I promise they are worth doing since they will make an enormous difference in how you feel. They have nothing to do with specific foods or what you can or can't eat; rather they focus on your style of eating. There are sound biochemical and psychological reasons for all six of them. In brief, they are:

Eat regular meals
Vary your diet
No late meals
No large meals
Prepare in advance
Enlist help

1. *Eat Regular Meals*. This sounds so simple and obvious, but it's one of the first things I impress on my patients and it can take real work—at first. By regular meals I mean that you should eat probably three times a day—at the same or nearly the same time each day. It doesn't matter what your schedule is. I've had as patients airline employees who are on erratic schedules, people who work night shifts, entertainers who get up at noon. It doesn't matter what your schedule is. What does matter is that shortly after you get up, whatever time that is, you have your first meal. Four or five hours later you should have a second meal and usually five or six hours after that, have your final meal of the day.

Eating regular meals is absolutely crucial for two reasons. First you need to supply your body with a steady source of energy throughout the day. Many of my patients who feel tired and irritable eat sporadically. They'll skip breakfast, grab something quick and not particularly nourishing for lunch, and then binge with a late dinner. Over a period of time they've become ever more reliant on quick fixes throughout the day, including coffee and sweets. That's because their bodies are desperate for energy, and they've learned that a quick fix will help. When they've gone without food for six, seven, or eight hours, their blood sugar drops and they feel weak, irritable, and fatigued. Coffee or sweets or even a cigarette will send their blood sugar soaring, and they feel temporarily better. Of course, we've seen how counterproductive these quick fixes are and how they lead to vague symptoms as well as future illness.

The second reason to eat regular meals each day is that it's a first step toward improving your eating habits. By providing your body with a steady source of energy-producing food throughout the day, you'll find it much easier to fight any cravings to indulge in caffeine, sugar, or cigarettes. You'll simply feel stronger. People who eat irregular meals think that they lack willpower when they can't stick to a diet. But I believe that irregular eating can affect their physiology to such a degree that it determines their psychology. Irregular eaters are starving themselves sporadically, and their bodies insist on overeating or overindulging when they finally get a chance.

Eating regularly of course means no skipping meals. Even if all you want is a piece of cold chicken, some crackers, and some fruit, it's far better than nothing. Going without a meal is setting yourself up for trouble. Behavior therapist Gordon Ball studied the eating patterns of rats, and found that the amount eaten at a meal is related not to the size of the previous meal, but to the interval between meals. A long interval means bigger amounts. If you give a rat his whole day's ration at one time, his stomach and intestines expand, he absorbs his food 40 percent faster, and he becomes fatter, calorie for calorie, than a rat who is eating regular meals of regular size. Researchers think this same pattern holds true for people.

2. *Vary Your Diet.* It amazes me sometimes how unvarying our diets can become. Some of my patients eat the same lunch five times a week and the same dinner as many times. It's easy to see how this happens. If you have a favorite meal you think is nutritious, low in calories, and easy to prepare or buy, you tend to eat it

often. I had one woman patient who lunched on cottage cheese and peaches every day for months on end! I think an every-other-day approach is good and simple; that is, rotating two different breakfasts and two different lunches if that's convenient.

It's important to avoid eating the same foods day after day and to try to eat as many different kinds as you can. There are three reasons for this.

For one thing, the more varied your diet, the better your chances of covering all your nutritional bases. Even though you're going to begin taking vitamin-mineral supplements next week, you can't count on getting all your nutrients from them. A varied diet will provide you with at least a good source of these nutrients.

A varied diet is also more likely to satisfy your hunger. When you eat the same foods all the time, you tend not to even notice what you're eating. It's just too boring. After eating the identical lunch five times in a row, you hardly feel as if you've had lunch. You're more likely to begin thinking about a snack as the day wears on. You may also feel as if you're punishing yourself by eating the same foods all the time. Eventually you might feel an overwhelming urge to rebel and have a hot-fudge sundae.

There's one more reason for varying your diet. I do a lot of work with my patients on food allergies. Many of them have developed allergies to a number of foods in their diet, and this happens most frequently when they eat the same things all the time. In most cases, these allergies are subtle. Patients don't break out in hives. But they may develop vague symptoms that they would never connect to a food allergy. These symptoms can include itching, fatigue, dizziness, blurred vision, headaches, excessive hunger, irritable-bowel syndrome, frequent colds, and sore throats. We're not dealing with food allergies in this book. Nonetheless, it has been my experience that eating a varied diet will help you avoid a tendency to develop food allergies. And by the way, if you suspect that you may be allergic to certain foods, you should see an allergist for tests. Since the most common food allergens are in wheat and dairy products, you could try eliminating first wheat then dairy foods to see if your symptoms are relieved.

3. *No Late Meals*. Research has demonstrated that, for reasons that aren't clear, people who eat meals late at night tend to gain weight even though they may be eating the same number of calories at the time as people who eat earlier in the evening. I've always recommended that my patients avoid late meals. For one thing, if they delay eating until late in the evening, they tend to be more hungry and to overeat. They're also sometimes too tired to prepare a good nutritious meal, and they simply eat whatever is fastest and easiest.

I suggest that you eat dinner no later than 8:00 P.M. if you are on a typical nine-to-five work schedule. I find that if I eat later than eight o'clock, I usually wake up at four in the morning. I thought this was an idiosyncratic reaction until I began to ask my patients about their meal and sleep schedules. It seems that many of those who had trouble going to sleep or who woke in the middle of the night were also eating late meals. As fatigue is one reason you tend to overeat, you can see that losing sleep because you've had a late meal can encourage you to overeat the next day.

4. *No Large Meals*. Naturally, if you have worked at weight control in the past, you are used to limiting your food intake and you avoid large meals. I find that if you follow the first three principles and eat a varied diet at regular times and don't eat late, you'll have no trouble avoiding large meals. People tend to eat too much when they've gone too long without food. So if you're eating regularly, you'll feel satisfied and will eat a reasonable amount at each meal.

Aside from caloric intake there's another reason to avoid large meals. Eating a large amount of food at one time seems to affect your metabolism. It will make you feel more tired, more fatigued, and more moody. Under those conditions you'll be more likely to ignore your principles of good nutrition.

How large is a large meal? Most people know when they're eating too much. It happens when you have some bread before dinner, soup, an appetizer, second helpings on some foods, and a dessert. I don't think you have to weigh your food in grams to know that a meal like this is too large. You should be satisfied with a vegetable, a protein, such as fish or chicken, and perhaps a salad. A cup of light soup can be a good beginning because it takes the edge off your hunger. A hearty soup can be a meal in itself. A piece of fruit is all you need for dessert.

5. *Prepare in Advance*. This is the most important principle of the New Nutrition. You can't follow any of the other principles unless you adhere to it.

I suggest that every evening, you think about the next day and what you're going to eat. Are you going out for lunch or dinner? Will you be eating at your desk? Should you bring something from home for lunch? Will you have to pick up something to prepare for dinner on the way home from work? What about snacks? Do you have enough fresh fruit in the house so you won't be tempted to dash out for cookies? Do you have the makings of a good breakfast?

It takes only a few minutes to think of these things ahead of time, and it's well worth it. So many of my patients have told me that the only times they have trouble with switching over to the New Nutrition is when they don't plan in advance. Bob K., a television cameraman, told me that he did well and felt great all during his first week of the New Nutrition. But about three weeks later he became very busy at work and neglected to plan ahead for lunch, which is the one meal he eats at the office—usually on the run. He'd been bringing soups and sandwiches from home, and was feeling full all afternoon, and thus could easily avoid the sweet snacks he used to depend on to last him until dinnertime. But for three days in a row he wound up grabbing lunch at the deli, and he just couldn't resist those little packaged cakes and potato chips that seemed to leap off the shelf while he was waiting in the busy deli lunch line. Each of these days, Bob found that he was starving by the time he got home for dinner, and it took all his self-control to avoid an afternoon sweet. He's back to planning his lunches, and pleased that he lost the extra fifteen pounds he had gained since college.

6. *Enlist Help*. Many people are secret dieters. They approach diets this way because they've often failed in the past, and they don't want to endure the public humiliation of another failure. Even though the New Nutrition is not a diet in the traditional sense of the word, it's still a change in eating habits, and it's my belief that you should get all the help you can to stick with it. Most people find two things helpful in this regard: They get their families to change to the New Nutrition and they tell their friends and co-workers what they're doing.

Fortunately, the New Nutrition is an excellent program for the whole family. Because it's not a so-called diet with specific amounts of foods, there is no reason why everyone in your household can't join you in your new eating habits. If you have children, they can only benefit from the New Nutrition. Studies have shown that many American children are malnourished because of all the empty calories they consume. A child will benefit as much as you from improved nutritional habits, and throughout life he or she will be reducing the risks of developing the same chronic diseases that you are avoiding. A child or a teenager might eat larger portions than an adult, but the foods can be the same. Many of my patients have found that they can control their weight and improve their nutrition if the whole family eats the same diet.

The only difficulty that some patients have reported is getting their children to go without sweets, but I have some suggestions for dealing with this problem later in this chapter.

Your family can be a major source of support, but your friends and co-workers can be too. My patients find that it's extremely useful to tell other people what they're trying to do. There's a great deal of interest today in nutrition, and many patients have told me that their friends and co-workers respond with great curiosity and encouragement when they explain their change in eating habits. You don't need to be a fanatic about this; it's counterproductive to rage against brownies and potato chips at an office party. But it's perfectly appropriate to tell someone who offers you a piece of fudge cake that you can't eat it. If they press you further, tell them about the New Nutrition.

Putting the New Nutrition into Practice

This Makeover week takes more advance preparation than most, depending on your current habits. If you are already eating reasonably well, you may simply have to do some extra shopping. In addition, if you're eating a poor diet, you may have to get rid of some of the foods around the house so they won't tempt you. In either case, you'll have to think about what you're going to eat in the week ahead. You don't have to plan every meal, but you do have to make sure that there will be something to eat for breakfast every day; that if you eat lunch at the office, you can either buy something nourishing or bring it from home; and that there will be nutritious food on hand to prepare for dinner so that you don't just grab something when you're too tired or hungry to eat what you should.

When you read the next section, keep a pad and

pencil handy. As you get ideas from these sections, jot down notes for food shopping. Do your shopping before the week begins. Most patients tell me that they find it useful to shop on the weekend for the week to come. Remember that you must plan ahead.

The Principles of the New Nutrition

The major goal of the New Nutrition is to shift the emphasis of your diet. You don't have to eat anything strange or in peculiar combinations or quantities. This is a nutritional program that you should be able to live with for the rest of your life.

There are three components to your diet: fat, protein, and carbohydrate. You need to eat all three to be properly nourished, but the question is, in what proportions. The following table shows in what proportions people generally do eat these components and in what proportions they should be eating them.

	Conventional Diet	New Nutrition Goals
Carbohydrate	46%	58%
Protein	12%	12%
Fat	42%	30%

You can see just by looking at the table you need to increase your carbohydrates and decrease your fats. Many people have already decreased the amount of fat they eat; but if you eat a great deal of meat, for example, you may have to work on decreasing protein too.

In keeping with these general goals, here are the more

specific goals of the New Nutrition that you should be working on this week.

1. *Eat Less Fat.* Fat is the most concentrated source of calories in your diet. It has 9 calories per gram, while both protein and carbohydrates have 4 calories per gram. You need fat to carry on your metabolic processes, but only the equivalent of one tablespoon per day—far less than is consumed by the average American.

As most people know, a diet rich in fat and cholesterol puts you at risk for heart disease, our nation's number one killer. Coronary heart disease is due to arteriosclerosis, which is a slow, progressive degeneration of the large arteries that begins early in life but rarely produces symptoms until middle age. In many cases the disease is undetected until the first heart attack, which is often fatal.

A high-fat diet has also been linked to two cancers that are major killers among Americans—cancer of the colon and breast cancer. The Japanese, who ate little fat of any kind until recently, when their diet became more "Westernized," have been largely free of these two cancers. One study of Seventh Day Adventists shows that if they ate meat, a component of a high-fat diet, they were two to three times more likely to develop colon cancer than those who ate a vegetarian diet their entire lives.

Reducing the fat in your diet may be the single most important step you can take toward better health and longer life. But it's not easy because so many foods we like contain fat, especially "convenience foods" that do not require preparation; for example, cheese. You'll have to work to reduce your fat intake, but it's well worth the trouble, and it should be the highest priority of your nutrition improvement week.

Here are some steps you can take to reduce the fat in your diet:

• **Eat less dairy food.** This will cut down on your cholesterol as well as your fat intake. Most people should cut their dairy-product intake in half; many people have twenty-four servings per week and should be having about twelve. Many people think that dairy products contain mainly protein when in fact they contain mostly fat. One of the quickest ways to cut down on dairy fat is to switch to low-fat or nonfat products. Some recent studies have shown that skim milk is not only low in fat, it also helps control cholesterol levels. Use skim milk instead of whole milk, low-fat yogurt instead of whole-milk yogurt, and low-fat cheeses. Most hard cheese contains more saturated fat than beef! Cottage cheese, pot cheese, farmers' cheese, and part-skim mozzarella and ricotta are good low-fat cheeses to substitute.

• **Eat less beef and pork.** Many people have already cut down on red meat, and this is all to the good. Though the beef industry claims that now it is breeding cattle with less fat, there is still a great deal of fat in an average serving of red meat. Most of us think that red meat is a great source of protein, but in fact a porterhouse steak has more fat in it than protein by weight. I think you should try to limit your red-meat intake to no more than two servings per week. You should eliminate organ meats, including liver, sweetbreads, and brains, which are very high in fat, except for an occasional serving. When you do have red meat, trim as much of the fat as possible before cooking.

• **When you cook meat, always drain off the fat before serving.** If, for example, you're cooking ground beef for spaghetti sauce, don't add extra fat for the browning—the meat will brown nicely in its own fat—and when the meat is brown, drain off every bit of extra fat in the pan. The fat has already done its job of flavoring the meat. Do the same with all other cooked meats, including chicken.

• **Eat more poultry,** but try to eat only white meat. The dark meat of chicken is the fattiest. Remove the skin from the chicken and any visible fat.

• **Change from butter or hard margarine** (made with

hydrogenated oil) **to soft tub margaine** (made with unhydrogenated oil).

• **Eliminate fried foods from your diet.** They contain too much fat. Broil, poach, bake, roast, steam, or barbecue (with a sugar-free sauce) instead. You can sometimes sauté foods, but should do so with very little fat. Most recipes call for double the fat you need. Use a nonstick pan and just a little bit of corn or olive oil with some broth added to it for a low-fat sauté.

• **Avoid commercial baked items.** We already know that they're loaded with sugar. Also they are often made with saturated fats. Don't buy any that just say "vegetable oil" on the label, or that specify they are made with coconut or palm oil or with animal fat. If you bake, use a polyunsaturated margarine for the fat in the recipe.

• **Make your own salad dressings.** Most recipes use an oil-to-vinegar ratio of three to one, but you can make a fine dressing with a reverse ratio, especially if you use a good flavorful vinegar like Italian balsamic vinegar. You can also make an excellent dressing with low-fat yogurt mixed in the blender with fresh herbs, like dill or basil, some minced garlic, and fresh-ground pepper. If you're using a dressing with oil in it, do so sparingly; it doesn't take much to coat a salad if you mix it well.

2. *Eat More Complex Carbohydrates.* Complex carbohydrates are available in starchy vegetables, whole-grain bread, unrefined cereals, brown rice, beans, and whole-wheat pasta. They should comprise over half your total calories.

Carbohydrates are not fattening—a five-ounce potato has about 110 calories, while five ounces of steak contains 500 calories. Moreover, natural unrefined carbohydrates, which are contained in whole grains, beans, fruits, and vegetables, are the only nutrients not linked to any leading killer diseases. If you increase your intake of these complex carbohydrates, you'll also be increasing your intake of vitamins, minerals, and trace nutrients, and at the same time, you'll be cutting down on your urge to eat calorie-rich fats and sweets.

Carbohydrates are also helpful in stabilizing blood sugar. They are digested slowly and help prevent dramatic highs and lows in blood sugar. They can also help you avoid binges because they fill your physical and psychological cravings for food. They actually fill you up better than any other food. A plate of pasta can not only satisfy your desire for a full meal, it also has fewer calories than a chicken dinner or a tuna salad.

Also, carbohydrates help control your appetite, as I explained earlier, by elevating your level of brain serotonin, which reduces carbohydrate craving. If you limit your carbohydrate intake, as some diets recommened you do, you won't be satisfying the body's need for them and you'll constantly feel hungry. This condition can be regarded as a carbohydrate hunger and, once satisfied, it will stop.

3. *Increase the Fiber in Your Diet.* By increasing carbohydrate consumption, you'll automatically be increasing the fiber in your diet, something most of us need to do. In March 1985, Health and Human Services Secretary Margaret Heckler predicted that if Americans increased their consumption of dietary fiber and lowered their use of fats, colon cancer could be reduced by 30 percent, saving 20,000 lives a year. In addition, fiber can help lower cholesterol and possibly prevent the development of heart disease. On a more immediate level, dietary fiber has a stabilizing effect on the blood sugar and can help prevent those periods of tiredness, irritability, fatigue, and moodiness. Additionally, increased fiber in the diet is the treatment of choice for chronic constipation.

Dietary fiber is the part of plant foods that the human body cannot digest. There are two kinds of fiber: that found primarily in fruits, vegetables, and dried beans, and that found in cereals and breads. Only the fiber from cereals and breads increases the bulk in the digestive system, and these seem the best for our purposes.

There are no official guidelines on how much fiber we should eat. The typical American diet contains an average of 15 to 20 grams of fiber a day. Most researchers advise that this amount could be raised to 30 or 35 grams a day without harm.

I usually recommend that my patients supplement their diet with bran, beginning with a teaspoon of miller's wheat bran and a teaspoon of oat bran. If they have a tendency toward constipation, I advise them to increase these amounts slowly until they have regular bowel movements. This has never failed if the increases are done *slowly*. There is some evidence that bran may reduce the absorption of certain minerals such as calcium, zinc, and iron, so take these supplements separately from the bran.

Here are some ways to increase your carbohydrate—and fiber—intake:

• **Eat more whole grains.** You can introduce them slowly into your diet so that you won't irritate your digestive system. Buy whole-grain cereals, bread, and crackers. Read the labels carefully, since many products that at first glance seem to be "whole grain" in fact contain little whole-grain flour. One of the very best ways to incorporate whole grains into your diet is with an oatmeal breakfast. Oatmeal made from rolled oats (skip the instant kind—it doesn't save that much time) contains the most protein of any popular grain, and the rolling used in processing does the least damage to the nutrients. One researcher discovered that you can reduce your risk of coronary heart disease by 20 percent just by eating oatmeal or an oat-bran muffin every morning and a half-cup of cooked beans at every lunch. The water-soluble fiber slows the production of cholesterol, and may also speed up the removal of excess cholesterol from the blood.

• **Avoid refined carbohydrates.** Since you've cut out sugar you're probably doing this already. But refined carbohydrates are found in foods like white rice and white refined flour as well as in sweet baked goods. As discussed, even if these items are called "enriched," they're not providing you with essential nutrients and may in fact be robbing you of some. Substitute brown rice for white rice and eat whole-wheat, buckwheat, or soy pasta products instead of white refined pastas. These are some of the best natural ways to increase fiber intake.

• **Eat more fresh fruits and vegetables.** Fruits and vegetables fill you up and add fiber and water to your diet. Moreover, a type of fiber called pectin, which is found in some fruits and vegetables—including apples and carrots—has been shown to help lower blood levels of cholesterol. Fresh fruits should be your main snack foods. You should also try to have some fresh fruit in the morning with breakfast instead of always relying on juice, as juice doesn't contain the necessary fiber.

• **Eat more salads.** Make them a mainstay of your diet, particularly in the summer when you can create a meal out of a salad by using some tuna or shrimp or bits of meat. When you make a salad, don't throw away the outer leaves of the lettuce, unless they're spoiled, since they contain more calcium, iron, and vitamin A than the inner leaves.

• **Eat more root vegetables** like cabbage and yams. Potatoes, although they have a high glycemic index, are low in calories and fill you up. But you can't go overboard on the butter. Use a bit of low-fat yogurt, mixed with fresh chives or other fresh herbs, on a baked potato. Try boiled new potatoes cooked in their skins to preserve nutrients.

4. *Change Your Main Source of Protein.* Most of us get plenty of protein in our diets, but over the years the source has changed. We now get over 70 percent of our protein from animal and dairy products, and, as we've seen, these foods are too high in fat. We should be putting much more emphasis on low-fat products and vegetables.

Here's how you can shift the emphasis of your protein source:

• **Eat more fish.** The average American eats about 12 pounds of fish each year, contrasted with 165 pounds of red meat. Seafood is low in saturated fat and high in protein. In fact, it's the best possible source of low-fat protein. Even seafood thought to be high in cholesterol—shrimp, crab, and lobster—contains less of it per serving than an egg. Not only that, recent research has shown that fish oil contains substances called omega-3 fatty acids that are very effective in lowering cholesterol. In general, the fattier the fish, the more omega-3s; salmon heads the list. Just be sure not to fry fish or add fatty condiments like tartar sauce, which will raise the fat content of your fish meal considerably.

• **Get more protein from soy.** Studies have shown that the cholesterol levels of people whose protein comes totally from soy—soy flour or textured soy protein—decrease consistently. Soy flour can be added to oatmeal, casseroles, hamburgers, meat loaf, and other foods. Fresh soybeans can be eaten in salads or as a side dish.

Tofu is an excellent source of soy protein. In fact, it's the basis of what my patients call "Dr. Giller's tofu shake." This shake is extremely popular with my patients as a complete breakfast. It's high in protein and low in calories, and it tastes delicious. You simply take one quarter of a cake of soft or firm tofu; one ripe banana, about one-half cup of crushed ice, one-half cup water, and mix together in the blender until smooth.

You can vary the recipe by using fresh or frozen berries (unsugared, of course), a dash of vanilla or almond flavoring, or even some oat bran to add fiber. I highly recommend that you try the shake, which is especially good in the summer when you may not feel like having a hot cereal like oatmeal for breakfast.

• Get some of your protein from dried beans and peas. You can use lentils, chick peas, and dried beans and peas in soups and casseroles. They will fill you up and keep your blood sugar on an even keel.

• Enlarge your repertoire of meatless meals that use low-fat cheeses and soy protein. Stir-fried vegetables with slices of tofu, and meatless lasagna made with low-fat cheese are two good protein dishes that are low in fat.

5. *Cut Down on Salt.* Everyone needs some salt, or sodium chloride, in their diets, but most people get far too much. The excess amount of salt in the American diet has been identified as a contributing factor to high blood pressure, kidney damage, premenstrual water retention and swelling, ringing in the ears, and heart disease.

A teaspoon of salt contains approximately 2,000 milligrams of sodium, a level considered within the safe range (1,100 to 3,300 milligrams) by the Food and Nutrition Board of the National Academy of Sciences. But current estimates of the daily sodium intake by most adults range from 2,300 milligrams to 6,900 milligrams—which means that some individuals get all the salt they need for a week in one day.

It isn't just the salt you add from the shaker that makes your daily consumption far too high—it's the salt in most prepared foods that you may not be aware you are consuming. While I advise my patients to cut down on salt by banning the salt shaker and avoiding processed foods, it is possible to lower the salt content of canned or processed food by rinsing it with water for up to three minutes. This will get rid of much of the salt, but the other nutrients won't be lost. Rinsing reduces the sodium content of green beans by more than 40 percent, of canned tuna by nearly 85 percent, and of cottage cheese by 63 percent.

If you cut down on salt, apparently you'll lose your taste for it, according to researchers at the University of Pennsylvania who report that "long-term reduction in dietary sodium alters the taste for salt." I've found that patients who are on a salt-restricted diet prefer less salty foods after a time, and discover that the amount of salt they consumed earlier makes food "too salty." If you cut back on salt for only a short time, however, you will crave it; it's the long-term reduction that changes your taste buds so you can appreciate the natural flavor of food.

Even though it's sold in health food stores, sea salt has the same effect as regular table salt. When you're reading labels at the supermarket, here's what to avoid:

Salt
Sodium chloride
Monosodium glutamate
Baking Soda
Baking Powder
Any additive that contains sodium
   as part of its identification

6. *Avoid Chemical Additives.* It is becoming increasingly clear that chemicals added to food for preserving, coloring, and flavoring are implicated in many diseases, (arthritis, migraine headaches, colitis, cancer, mental problems, and hyperactivity, to name a few). For unknown reasons, these chemicals can cause individuals to develop irritation and inflammation in weak systems or organs of the body.

Effective nutritional treatment of many ailments can begin with the elimination of foods that contain chemical additives. Unfortunately, because the food industry has ignored the problem, these foods may include many canned goods and bottled drinks and some frozen products. Whenever you buy something that is not fresh, *read the label carefully.* You will probably be surprised at the number of chemicals you are consuming. While attempts have been made to remove some of the chemicals from food, many of those in use today are still undergoing tests to determine if they are safe. My suggestion is not to wait for government to do it for you, but to begin eliminating food additives from your diet now. By substituting additive-free foods for a feast of chemicals, you will be doing yourself a great favor.

Some common foods containing additives are canned goods; processed meats such as bacon, hot dogs, luncheon spreads, etc.; dry cereals; soft drinks; packaged desserts; foods that have been precooked, fabricated, altered, or are imitations. Even Grade A meat is no longer additive-free. The Food and Drug Administration (FDA) reports that fully 80 percent of the meat we eat comes from animals fed with tetracycline or other antibiotics. This includes cattle, hogs, sheep, chickens, and turkeys.

Antibiotics enable animals to gain weight quickly, which permits breeders to bring them to market sooner. Yet these antibiotics cause the bacteria in animals' systems to become immune to the germ-killing powers of antibiotics. Humans could then ingest the diseased animals and this may cause severe illness. Additionally, some scientists fear that this practice will spur the development of drug-resistant germs that could pose more hazards to human health.

Does this sound far-fetched? It's not. Instances of such chain reactions have been documented. An epidemic of *Salmonella typhimurium* food poisoning in England was attributed to beef that had been grown on medicated feed. The epidemic caused illness in some six hundred people. Six died. Conventional drug treatment was not successful in treating the afflicted. British farmers are no longer allowed to use the same antibiotics in animal feed that physicians prescribe for humans, and although the FDA is considering similar regulations, no action is expected in the near future.

In their search to find ways to increase weight gain in livestock, cattlemen have hit upon hormones. One is diethylstilbestrol (DES), a synthetic female hormone. DES is known to be the cause of a rare vaginal cancer in women whose mothers were treated with DES during pregnancy twenty years earlier. Many young women have died. Additionally, it has been shown that DES produces cancer in laboratory animals. Cattlemen are now required to remove DES from the diet of their cattle fourteen days before slaughter, presumably to allow the hormone to pass through the edible tissue and be excreted.

However, many environmentalists doubt that cattlemen abide by this restriction. The *Environment Action Bulletin* reports that twenty-one other countries, including Argentina and Australia, the world's largest beef producers, have banned all uses of DES. Yet it is still allowed in the United States.

Few suspected cancer-related agents in our food have achieved more notoriety than sodium nitrate and sodium nitrite, chemicals which exist naturally in some foods in minute amounts. They are used in large amounts to preserve ham, pastrami, corned beef, bacon, frankfurters, bologna, and other luncheon meats. Under certain conditions, nitrates and nitrites combine with amines to form dangerous nitrosamines, which can cause malignant tumors. It's virtually impossible to avoid amines, as they are found in meat proteins, cigarette smoke, beer, wine, many patent medicines, and prescription drugs.

Nitrates and nitrites do prevent the growth of botulism bacteria, which can cause deadly food poisoning, but the FDA and even some meat packers admit that this function is comparatively minor, since improved refrigeration techniques negate the importance of this treatment, except for canned ham.

So why are they still used? For cosmetic reasons, so the meat looks red and fresh. These chemicals cause the meat to retain its reddish color, which would be lost without them.

Nutrition Tips from Makeover Veterans

Because I don't give my patients a specific diet to improve nutrition, I've found over the years that they have devised quite ingenious solutions to their nutritional dilemmas, and have shared their ideas with me. I've collected the best of their tips and will list them here. I think you'll find them helpful.

• One of my patients is always in too much of a rush in the morning to have breakfast, so he simply packs something the night before and brings it to the office to eat at his desk. He often has an apple and some low-fat cheese, or a bran muffin and an orange.

• Use plain, low-fat yogurt instead of sour cream in sauces. Just add cornstarch—one tablespoon per cup of yogurt—to keep it from separating when heated.

• Get rid of leftovers quickly. One woman told me that if she has little bits of leftover food around, she tends to eat them, but she has learned to toss them out. Another patient said he keeps a container for leftovers in the fridge, puts everything in it, then feeds the contents to the dog. Another person gives leftovers from dinner parties to guests as they leave.

• Ban tempting foods from your house. I have always done this and strongly suggest that my patients do so. If it's not there, you can't eat it. Many people buy cookies or candy "for the kids," but wind up eating most of it themselves. Neither you nor the kids need it and you'll have no trouble resisting if it's not there in the first place.

• Don't shop when you're hungry. Many people have heard this, but one patient emphasized how important it is. He always used to shop for dinner on his way home from work. But he would always be starving, so he would often buy a treat to eat on the way home, and too much food for his evening meal. Now he tries to shop on weekends and figure out in advance what he wants to eat so he can have everything ready. When he gets home, he can quickly prepare a nutritious meal and satisfy his hunger.

• If you go to a buffet dinner, always eat sitting down and be aware of what you are eating. One of my patients said that because she didn't sit down at a buffet dinner, she didn't think she was having much to eat. It was only later, when she added everything up, that she realized she had consumed a large quantity of canapés high in fat.

• When you order a sandwich in a deli or coffee shop, specify the kind of bread that you would like. Few restaurants offer real whole-wheat bread; the bread usually contains 20 percent whole-wheat flour, and the rest is white flour with caramel coloring. Rye or pumpernickel is a good bet. Fresh French bread or Italian bread, although white, is usually free of the thirty or more dough conditioners, bleaches, and preservatives that are in most pre-sliced breads.

• In restaurants order all sauces and salad dressings, which are high in fat, on the side. Then you can control how much you use. If the waiter says he can't bring the sauce separately, this is a sign that the dish was precooked, frozen, and then reheated—or that the quality is less than you would expect.

• Chinese, Indian, and Japanese restaurants are good

choices for healthy dining, since these cuisines are based on grains and vegetables, with meat and fish as supplements. You can order traditional dishes that use very little fat, butter, cream, or cheese. One of my patients had to eat out with clients frequently, and had trouble ordering healthy food until he began suggesting one of these three kinds of restaurants. Most of his clients didn't object; in fact, they welcomed the change of pace.

• In an American restaurant, ask for plain grilled fish or chicken. In a steak house, consider ordering a double shrimp cocktail as a main course.

• When everybody else is ordering dessert, don't forget to use the line "I'm prediabetic" if the situation is making you uncomfortable. This will stop everybody urging you to "go ahead—you're so thin anyway."

• If you're going to a cocktail party, eat beforehand. Having something in your stomach will make it easier to pass up those fatty hors d'oeuvres—and the drinks.

• At a dinner party, if the hostess doesn't have club soda when you ask for it, tell her you have some in your car and would she mind if you drank that?

A simple, healthful daily diet that incorporates the principles of the New Nutrition might include:

BREAKFAST: 2 oz. protein (preferably low fat)
(or a tofu shake which combines both)
1 fruit
Herbal tea

LUNCH: 4 oz. protein, preferably low fat, such as fish or chicken
1 cup salad
½ cup vegetables

DINNER: 4 oz. protein, preferably low fat, such as fish
           or chicken
        2 cups salad
        1½ cups vegetables

SNACKS: Raw vegetables, fruit
        Optional: 1 slice bread daily

Week Four:
Vitamins and Minerals, the New Nutrition Supplements

You're nearly halfway through your Medical Makeover, and I'm happy to tell you that this will be your easiest week. Now that you're enjoying life without caffeine and sugar, reaping the benefits of good nutrition, and taking your antistress and antilow-blood-sugar supplements, you should be feeling better than you have in years. If you're like most of my patients, by Week Four of the Makeover, you're learning how *satisfying* it can feel to be in charge of your good health, to wake up in the morning with energy and enthusiasm. As Margaret D., an assistant buyer at a major department store, told me, "This is no longer a program for me; it's a way of life. If I want to feel healthy, which is what I want, there's no other option. For me, feeling good is its own reward." I hope that by now you feel that way too.

This Week's Goal

This week is easy because you're not unlearning an old pattern of behavior, you're simply learning something new. And it's easy and even fun. First, I'm going to convince you why you need vitamins, tell you what they can do for you in the short and long terms. Then you'll take a quiz that will help you determine exactly which nutritional supplements you should be taking. By the end of the week you will have established a regime of vitamin and mineral supplementation that will go a long way toward filling any nutritional gaps in your diet.

Vitamins and Minerals: Snake Oil or Sensible?

Vitamins are organic food substances that are absolutely essential for the maintenance of life: They are necessary for normal growth, metabolism, and our physical and mental well-being. Found only in living things, these nutrients must be obtained in the diet because the body does not manufacture them. Vitamins do not provide energy directly to the body, but they are necessary for complicated chemical reactions that turn food into energy and structure. From vitamins our bodies make the substances that are vital for the healthy functioning of body and—as we've learned in the last several decades mind.

For example, for the brain to get energy from blood sugar, at least a dozen different chemical reactions must take place. At each step, one or more vitamins are necessary.

Minerals work in tandem with vitamins and, like vitamins, act as catalysts for numerable biological reactions within the body and brain. Unlike vitamins, minerals are found in both organic and inorganic matter. When they are in the soil in which a particular vegetable or fruit is grown, they become part of the structure of that plant and are absorbed when the plant is eaten. Plants use minerals for their own internal metabolism. It is thought that mineral deficiencies in humans may be even more common than vitamin deficiencies.

Minerals have two general functions in the body: building and regulating. Minerals are important constituents of bones, teeth, tissues, muscles, blood, and nerve cells. They also help regulate many biological reactions, such as heartbeat, nerve responses, blood clotting, balancing internal fluids, utilizing oxygen, and aiding digestion and metabolism in general.

It's the unusual consumer who's not at least a little confused about vitamins and minerals. On the one hand, there's a whole industry that has grown up with lightning speed to convince people that they need vitamins. In 1972 the vitamin business earned about $500 million in sales; in 1988 it is expected to earn about $3.5 billion. About 44 percent of us take at least one vitamin per day, but most of us aren't exactly sure why or what for. On the other hand, we often read some medical writers or hear doctors say that we are really simply producing "the most expensive urine in the world." I think Arlene K., who works as a publicist for an art-book publisher, was typical of the average confused vitamin consumer. When she came to see me, she was taking a multivitamin plus two or three additional supplements that would vary depending on what she had just read about a particular vitamin or mineral helping your skin, your hair, your digestion, your resistance to infection, or whatever. Arlene told me that she was never really convinced that these vitamins made much difference, but they seemed like a good "health insurance policy."

Through my experiences with my patients, and because of the latest research on vitamins and minerals, I've become convinced that supplements are an essential part of complete nutrition. It's an extremely rare individual with an extremely rare diet—and I've never encountered such a person in years of computerized nutritional analyses of my patients—who doesn't need some vitamin supplementation.

I do not consider my program megavitamin therapy. I prescribe optimum replacement dosages for deficiencies that are the result of poor nutrition, bad habits, special needs, or that will counteract symptoms that my patients experience. Megavitamin therapy should be attempted only under the care of a doctor. Treating yourself with larger doses than recommended here can be dangerous. Vitamin replacement or supplementation, on the other hand, is an effort to ensure that your body is getting the necessary vitamins to allow daily metabolic processes to function efficiently and prevent the onset of future chronic diseases. Personal vitamin supplementation dosages are what you are going to start this week.

What to Expect from Vitamins and Minerals

Vitamins and minerals are not miracle substances. They only help problems that are brought on by a specific deficiency.

Vitamin and mineral supplements, when used in conjunction with a nutritious diet, simply ensure that you are giving your particular body the tools it needs to **achieve optimum helath.** It sometimes takes weeks for the real effects of the supplements to be felt because it takes that long for them to affect your metabolism. But some of my patients report an almost immediate improvement that they ascribe to vitamins. For example, the antistress formula in Week One helps you cope better immediately, and the chromium you began to take in Week Two probably had a swift effect on your sweet cravings. Many people report the disappearance of minor symptoms; for example, the alleviation of leg cramps with calcium supplementation.

But for some of you, it probably won't be until the end of your Makeover that you really benefit from your vitamin-mineral program. At the same time, the supplementation program will begin to help you improve your metabolism right from the very beginning and make it easier to follow through with the rest of the Makeover. In fact, the program will help strengthen you, so that when you begin the alcohol, the smoking, and stress-management weeks, you'll be in the best possible condition to deal with what, for some people, are the most difficult weeks.

Finally I want to stress that vitamins and minerals are not substitutes for good nutrition. They must be used in combination with a well-balanced diet. That's why the nutrition week precedes the vitamin week. Vitamins are facilitators, but food is where the process of nutrition starts. There is no point in taking supplements if you are not eating properly; it's like putting high-performance oil in a car with no gas.

Vitamins: How Much Is Enough?

If you ate a diet consisting of precise amounts of purified fats, proteins, and carbohydrates that were administered to you in exactly the quantities recommended by the most up-to-date nutritionist, you would not flourish. These substances are macronutrients. Essential to sustain life, they can't do so on their own. In addition to macronutrients, we need to consume micronutrients—vitamins and minerals—that act as catalysts and facilitate energy production of the macronutrients.

A well-known observation that linked disease to the lack of a specific food was made in 1747 when it was discovered that there was a dramatic improvement in scurvy cases among British seamen if they ate oranges and lemons. Eventually the navy ordered an ounce of lemon juice per day per man, and it was claimed that this preventive measure doubled British manpower at sea. It also inspired the nickname "limeys" for British sailors.

The early work with vitamins set the approach that

would be followed for years to come. The research focused on severe deficiencies, those serious enough to cause disease and even death. While this approach was valid at the time, it inspired an attitude toward vitamins and minerals that was not always enlightened. Once it was realized that certain amounts of vitamins and minerals were needed to prevent certain diseases, researchers came to believe that if these amounts were provided, nutritional health could be assured. And the only reason to provide vitamins was if a person was diseased. Then the pendulum swung in the opposite direction, and people began to make extravagant claims for vitamins which were eventually disproved.

Today we are on a middle ground, with many people confused about the truth about vitamins. Because many doctors believe that we get adequate nutrition from a balanced diet, they are convinced that vitamins are unnecessary. If you don't have the sign of a severe vitamin deficiency, the thinking goes, then you don't need supplementation.

This approach to health and nutrition perpetuates several myths: that generally we eat a balanced diet with all the nutrients we need, that the Recommended Daily Allowances (RDAs) are adequate for all people, that we are biochemically so alike that we do not need varying amounts of vitamins and minerals, and that the deficiency state of a vitamin or mineral exists only when severe clinical symptoms—i.e., disease—are present.

What Vitamin "Deficiency" Means to You

Most of us think of vitamin deficiency as something that results in beriberi or rickets, or some rare disease that no one in the industrialized world gets anymore. We learned about these deficiencies in grammar school and feel quite complacent that we're protected against them.

This is a very unsophisticated view of vitamin-mineral deficiencies. As with all the other chronic diseases we have discussed, a vitamin deficiency doesn't show up overnight and it isn't a simple black or white issue. There are minor levels of deficiencies that can affect you in subtle ways every day of your life.

There are three levels of change that occur in your body when a vitamin or mineral is lacking. First, your stores of that vitamin are depleted. Second, there is a subtle change in metabolism that could cause minor symptoms of deficiency. And finally, only in the third stage is there evidence of classical clinical symptoms.

A study recently demonstrated these three stages. Volunteers were deprived of vitamin B_1. For five to ten days, no changes were discovered. Then, after ten days of depletion, there was evidence of changes in cellular metabolism. The classical signs of vitamin B_1 deficiency weren't seen until two hundred days after the vitamin was stopped, but during those two hundred days, even though there were none of the classical signs of B_1 deficiency, the volunteers experienced declining health and increased illness. They had vague symptoms, including loss of weight, loss of appetite, fatigue, insomnia, and increased irritability.

Osteoporosis is a disease that has received a lot of attention. Osteoporosis is due to a deficiency of calcium, and it results in brittle bones. In most cases, its worst effects aren't seen until a woman is in her fifties or sixties. Well, these women didn't develop osteoporosis overnight. I see young women patients every day who, I am sure, are developing osteoporosis. X rays would show no signs of the disease, and they have none of the clinical symptoms like frequent bone fractures. But they do have recurrent leg cramps or bleeding gums or peeling nails. These are early signs of calcium deficiency. If these women do not notice and treat the symptoms now, they will develop full-blown cases of osteoporosis in twenty years. That's why my personal vitamin-mineral dosage profile looks for early signs of minor deficiencies.

Perhaps the most famous case of marginal mineral deficiency involved Alberto Salazar, the marathon runner. His long-distance running performance was clearly declining and, despite a number of medical tests, no reason could be found. But on closer observation it was discovered that his iron stores were depleted. Normally if your iron stores are depleted, the first sign would be anemia, but it has recently been discovered that before you develop anemia, you might suffer from fatigue and reduced performance on exertion. When Salazar took iron supplements, his performance improved. If he were not a famous runner, but just a part-time athlete like so many people, his marginal deficiency would probably never have been discovered.

Obviously your body begins to react to a vitamin or mineral deficiency long before you develop the signs of any disease connected with that deficiency. If you are aiming for optimum health, you don't want to wait to develop clinical signs of a disease: You want your metabolism to function at a peak level all the time. There is evidence that even a marginal deficiency of a vitamin or mineral will contribute to the vague symptoms that we have discussed throughout the Makeover. Fatigue, lethargy, irritability, difficulty in concentrating, insomnia, and even a lowered resistance to infection and disease can all result from just a marginal deficiency. And though an average diet, or even a relatively poor diet, won't completely deprive our bodies of specific vitamins for extended periods of time, it certainly won't give us our optimum daily vitamin or mineral needs.

The Myth of the "Balanced Diet"

One of the biggest arguments against vitamin-mineral supplementation is that we get all the nutrients we need from the "average American diet." I wondered about the adequacy of my patients' diets, and so I began a program of computerized nutritional analysis. I would have my patients keep track of the foods they ate for two weeks. In a somewhat tedious process, they noted every single food, including the amount, that they consumed each day. Then a computer evaluated their diet for vitamins, minerals, fiber, carbohydrates, fat, cholesterol, protein, etc. Over a period of years and after testing several thousand people, including patients who are very health-conscious and make an effort to eat nutritiously, I have yet to see one whose diet is completely adequate in terms of the Recommended Daily Allowances of vitamins and minerals. Not only are they not getting sufficient vitamins and minerals to prevent deficiencies, they're not getting nearly enough for optimum health and well-being.

Many controlled studies have demonstrated what I found with my patients. In 1971 the first National Health and Nutrition Examination Survey—a four-year study—examined the diets of 28,000 people across the country. Despite the fact that the survey used very conservative standards, dramatic dietary deficiencies were found. More than 60 percent of the people tested, regardless of income level, showed at least one symptom of malnutrition. And remember, the nutritional standards were based on those devised to prevent serious deficiencies, not those devised to promote optimum health.

Countless other studies have had similar results. A 1978 study of fifteen thousand households found that things are getting worse rather than better: The household diets were even more deficient than those of the individuals who were studied in 1971. A 1985 study at the Beltsville Human Nutrition Center in Maryland followed the diets of twenty-eight young middle-class men and women for a year to determine the nutrient intake of adults who live at home and consume supposedly good diets. Daily intakes of zinc, copper, magnesium, calcium, and phosphorus were all found to be deficient. Even hospital diets, with the expert help of dietitians and nutritionists, can't seem to provide adequate nutrition. One study demonstrated that more than 75 percent of the patients in one hospital became malnourished over the course of their stay.

Why can't we get necessary nutrition from even a "healthy diet"? How did people live before vitamins? The fact is that before vitamin supplements, foods were much healthier and provided far more vitamins and minerals than today's diets. Food processing, among other things, strips our food of vitamins. Orange juice in a waxed container, for example, has lost about 20 percent of its vitamin C. Israeli scientists have found that an orange-banana mixture which is produced for infants loses 75 to 80 percent of its vitamin C through processing. Dr. Henry Schroeder, one of America's foremost authorities on the nutrient content of food, did vitamin-mineral studies on 730 common foods. He discovered that the canning of green vegetables, for example, destroys more than 50 percent of vitamins B_5 and B_6, and the canning of carrots destroys more than 70 percent of the cobalt. Freezing destroys over half the B vitamins of most foods. Freezing meat, for example, destroys 70 percent of vitamin B_5. The list of lost nutrients revealed by Dr. Schroeder's test is endless.

As we eat more and more processed foods, we lose more and more nutrients. In 1940, 10 percent of our foods were processed. In 1970 processed foods accounted for 50 percent of our diet. As women working outside the home becomes the rule rather than the exception, and processed foods become more palatable, and the microwave oven becomes nearly ubiquitous, we can assume that the figure will grow.

Processed foods encourage a new kind of malnutrition which has been called "overconsumptive undernutrition." They don't cause beriberi or rickets, but do contribute to our "civilized plagues," the major chronic diseases, including heart disease, cancer, diabetes, obesity, and the breakdown of the immune system. In 1971, Dr. Edith Weir of the U.S. Department of Agriculture estimated that if the diet of all Americans was brought up just to the level of the Recommended Daily Allowances (a minimal and, in the eyes of many, an inadequate level that we will discuss later), there would be major improvements in at least nineteen serious health problems and a half million lives would be saved annually.

"Fresh" foods are often not much more nutritious from a vitamin-mineral standpoint than processed foods are. Lettuce that's stored at room temperature loses 50 percent of its vitamin C just twenty-four hours after picking. If it's refrigerated, it loses the same amount in three days. Asparagus, broccoli, and green beans also lose 50 percent of their vitamin C in cold storage before they reach your grocer.

The ways in which we prepare food further robs it of nutrients. When a researcher actually tested the government's 1978 USDA tables that specify what nutrients are found in given foods, she found that in some cases the actual nutrients were only one third as much as had been specified. For example, the government tables say that seven ounces of spaghetti and sauce contain 8 milligrams of vitamin C, but the researcher discovered that the spaghetti and sauce she tested had only 1.2 milligrams. Eighty-five percent of the vitamin C was missing. It seems that we can't even count on getting the vitamins and minerals that are claimed to exist in certain foods.

"Enriched" foods, with vitamins and minerals added, are more a marketing device than a nutritional one. The body uses a combination of vitamins and minerals in its metabolic processes. For example, niacin, thiamine, riboflavin, pantothenic acid, pyridoxine, phosphorus, and magnesium are required to metabolize carbohydrates. Over half of these nutrients are lost when white flour is milled; a small percentage is put back and the bread is called "enriched." For the body to use this "enriched" bread, it has to steal nutrients from stored sources in various tissues in the body. Phosphorus, magnesium, pantothenic acid, and pyridoxine all have to be "stolen" in order for the body to metabolize the bread. These "robbed" tissues are left deficient. Over a period of time the "enriched" foods you eat can be starving your body of essential nutrients. It is obvious that most Americans are slowly and secretly developing deficiencies.

The Myth of the RDA

Now that it's clear that our diet lacks essential nutrients, how do we know what amounts of vitamins and minerals we should be getting? We are supposed to look at the RDAs. The RDAs are the Recommended Dietary Allowances of vitamins and minerals that the Food and Nutrition Board of the National Research Council has determined. The RDAs were developed during World War II when the government was concerned that the K rations issued to the troops would contain sufficient vitamins and minerals. The goal of the RDAs was to provide a guideline that would prevent large segments of the population from developing serious nutritional deficiencies. Supposedly, if we consume vitamins and minerals in the amounts indicated in the RDAs, we'll be fulfilling our nutritional needs. But it's generally recognized that the RDAs do not promote optimum health or, for some people, even minimal health. Indeed, there are many who are openly scornful of the RDAs.

Senator William Proxmire said, "The RDA standard is established by the Food and Nutrition Board of the National Research Council which is influenced, dominated, and financed in part by the food industry. It represents one of the most scandalous conflicts of interest in the federal government." He also summed up the RDAs as follows: "At best the RDA's are only a 'recommended' allowance at antediluvian levels designed to prevent some terrible disease. At worst they are based on the conflicts of interest and self-serving views of certain portions of the food industry. Almost never are they provided at levels to provide for optimum health and nutrition."

Linus Pauling, the Nobel Prizewinner, has argued against the validity of the dosages in the RDAs. He said, "The RDA for a vitamin is not the allowance that leads to the best of health for most people. It is, instead, only the estimated amount that for most people would prevent death or serious illness from vitamin deficiency. Values of the daily intake of the various vitamins that lead to the best of health for most people may well be several times as great, for the various vitamins, as the values of the RDA." He also makes the point that minimal vitamin intake can mean minimal health: ". . . no vitamin lack strikes overnight or in a day or two, in contrast to the quick manner of infectious diseases or foreign poisons. Many weeks, or even many months, are usually required for signs of a vitamin deficiency to appear. The cells continue to function, but at reduced efficiency due to lower enzyme levels. Then as they decline further or die, different tissues and organs will slowly be affected."

One of the problems with the RDAs is that the best way to arrive at more accurate and precise figures concerning nutritional needs would be out of bounds. Because of obvious ethical problems researchers can't withhold essential nutrients from people to see how they respond. So what they do is determine how much of a

certain vitamin a healthy person ingests as, for example,
they did with vitamin E. It was noted in a study that
apparently healthy adults ingested approximately 15 units
(technically called International Units, or IU) of vitamin
E every day. So this became the RDA standard for
vitamin E. Would these people have done better on
twenty? Were they as healthy as they could be? It
brings us back to the question of the definition of health.
Is it absence of disease or optimal functioning? We're
aiming, of course, for optimal functioning.

We do know that there are many examples in animal
studies where minimal levels of vitamins and minerals
have meant minimal health. For example, a study on
guinea pigs to determine how much vitamin C would
prevent scurvy revealed that the amount which would
prevent disease was ten times lower than the amount
that would optimize wound healing, promote growth
rate, and reduce recovery time after anesthesia. Dr.
Man-Li Yew suggested that on the basis of his research,
children may need much more vitamin C than previously
believed: "It appears that for young people the need is at
least 20 times higher than the accepted RECOMMENDED
Dietary Allowance. Individual needs vary over a wide
range, and the implications of these findings may be
much more widespread than just vitamin C itself." Numerous other studies have demonstrated that children
receiving higher than RDA dosages have increased growth
and health.

The RDAs don't really claim to be the ideal guideline
for everyone. In fact, the Food and Nutrition Board of
the National Academy of Sciences states specifically that
"RDA should not be confused with requirements." They
go on to specify the three major limitations of the RDAs:

1. They apply only to healthy people who, in our
stressful, polluted environment, are increasingly rare.
2. They guarantee a minimal level of nutrition.

3. It is very probable that even a healthy person will need greater amounts of certain nutrients than are specified by the RDAs because of his or her unique biochemical individuality. What is adequate for one individual may be sorely lacking for another. For example, some people do not absorb enough of a certain vitamin, and need to compensate by taking a supplement in order to get an adequate amount; others may not be able to convert the vitamin to the active form the body is able to utilize; the excessive intake of certain foods may make an otherwise adequate amount insufficient.

The RDAs don't take into account differences in age, life-style, environment, height, weight, occupation, temperament, emotional or physical stress, illness, metabolic problems, bad habits, activity levels, changes in weather, which can affect nutrient needs, or any medications you might be taking, all of which can have an effect on your nutritional needs.

Special groups of people who are more at risk for vitamin deficiencies than others include: infants, children who have poor eating habits or who are on weight-reduction diets, pregnant and lactating women, women on birth control pills, heavy smokers; people who take large doses of aspirin—such as arthritis sufferers—strict vegetarians, alcoholics, and elderly people.

It seems that nearly everybody falls into a special category. The RDAs were originally designed for healthy twenty-two-year-olds who do light labor. Not people who live in polluted cities. Not people who have stressful jobs. Not people like you and me.

Does this mean that we should ignore the RDAs? No, we should simply use them as a baseline, and, because we're aiming for optimal health, we factor in all the personal differences that are affecting our nutritional requirements, and we modify the RDAs to suit our unique needs.

Biochemical Individuality

One last concept helps explain why you may not be getting adequate vitamins and minerals—regardless of the RDAs or the fact that you don't have rickets or beriberi. It has to do with the fact that you and I are vastly different from each other.

You may fall asleep after one glass of wine while your friend can drink nearly a full bottle before feeling its effects. Though drugs are sometimes prescribed by body weight, we know that they affect people in widely differing ways that have nothing to do with body weight. We know that the hormone levels in two people of the same age can differ dramatically. As your body is unique in shape and size, so also it is unique in its nutritional needs. No two individual metabolisms are the same. These differences are referred to as "biochemical individuality."

Roger Williams, past president of the American Chemical Society, has documented thousands of differences among people, particularly in relation to their nutritional needs. In working with laboratory animals, for example, he discovered that some rats need forty times more vitamin A than others. He has proposed that many degenerative diseases are the end result of our ignorance of differing nutritional requirements: Some people live in a chronically deficient state that eventually leads to gout, arteriosclerosis, alcoholism, multiple sclerosis, muscular dystrophy, and mental depression. Concerning alcoholism, for example, he found that when rats in the laboratory were given a choice between alcohol and water, the animals whose diets were well fortified with vitamins and minerals preferred water while the ones on a deficient diet consumed more alcohol.

Dr. Linus Pauling found that vitamin C excretion varies by a factor of 16 from person to person, and that of vitamin B_6 by a factor of 35. This means that individual vitamin needs can vary by 3,500 percent! Even taking into consideration the fact that someone with an extremely high or an extremely low requirement would throw off the curve, this still indicates that relying on the RDAs to determine what your body needs is probably not accurate.

Obviously, with a potential for so much variation, it's crucial that vitamin dosages must be tailored to your unique personal needs as precisely as possible. Biochemical individuality means that you must look for clues in your behavior and sense of well-being, and in the way your particular body reacts to different supplements, in order to find your optimum vitamin-mineral supplement level. That's the purpose of our personalized supplement quizzes.

Preparing for the Week

Preparing for Week Four couldn't be easier. All you have to do is figure out your personal vitamin-mineral profile by taking the quiz beginning on page 174. Once you've figured out the doses you should be taking, all you need do is simply buy the vitamins.

You are already taking your basic antistress supplements. The multiple vitamin and mineral contains your basic protection. The antioxidants are helping you cope with stress, and the chromium is keeping your blood sugar stable. But now you need to know what other supplements are necessary for your unique biochemical makeup. I do not believe that there is one multivitamin and mineral supplement that is suitable for everybody, but the basic multiple I recommend is a starting point. Thereafter, needed supplements are added according to your responses to the following quizzes.

Your Personal Vitamin-Mineral Profile

No one can predict the precise dosages of various vitamins you should be taking to meet your unique needs. If it were possible to do this, the RDAs could be made effective for each individual. But here are some guidelines. The Basic Protection Dosage is shown right at the end of each vitamin-mineral description. I can't guarantee that these dosages are going to be optimal for you, but I can guarantee that they will be much better than the RDAs and will help you achieve the three-pronged goal of optimum health you're seeking.

I suggest that you get out a pad and pencil, and as you read through the list of vitamins, note what your personal recommended dosage is. At the same time, note if that vitamin should be taken all at once or in divided dosages. Your multivitamin is best taken at breakfast, and all of the vitamins, unless noted, should be taken with meals. Remember, as you're already taking a multivitamin, your final dosage of each vitamin should take into account the dosage you're getting in that multivitamin.

Please remember that this vitamin assessment is for people who are basically healthy, not for people suffering from disease. It is not a prescription, does not purport to treat any illness, and should not be used in place of medical treatment. If you are taking any medication, check with your doctor to be sure your vitamin regimen is appropriate. For example, if you take Accutane, you should avoid vitamin A.

Vitamins

Vitamin A

Vitamin A is necessary for the growth and repair of body tissues, for the health of the eyes, for fighting bacteria and infection. Because vitamin A plays an important role in protecting the mucous membranes of the body, including those in the nose, mouth, throat, and lungs, it can help protect us to some degree from the ravages of air pollution. Beta-carotene, a precursor form of vitamin A, is thought to be an especially effective antioxidant. Optimally, half of your total vitamin A dosage should be beta-carotene.

Good sources of vitamin A include carrots and fish oil as well as green leafy vegetables like beet greens, spinach, and broccoli. One carrot contains about 20,000 IU of vitamin A and a half pound of calf's liver contains about 70,000 IU.

Because vitamin A is fat-soluble, it can build up in the body. For adults, taking more than 85,000 IU per day of vitamin A can quickly become toxic. Symptoms of vitamin A toxicity include: headaches, dry skin, sore lips, diarrhea, hair loss, nausea, vomiting, and dizziness. Discontinuing the vitamin will cause the symptoms to disappear. If you notice any symptoms of vitamin A toxicity (and you shouldn't on the dosages I recommend), eliminate the vitamin temporarily, then resume taking it at a lower dosage.

For each question that applies to you, add the appropriate amount of vitamin A, not exceeding a total daily dosage of 25,000 IU. Vitamin A may be taken at one time and with other vitamins or minerals at any meal.

1. **Do you have trouble seeing in medium-dim light or have poor night vision? (10,000 IU)** _____
2. **Do you drink more than two alcoholic beverages per day? (10,000 IU)** _____
3. **Are you prone to frequent upper respiratory infections? (10,000 IU)** _____
4. **Do you suffer from acne? (25,000 IU)** _____
5. **Are you a smoker? (10,000 IU)** _____
6. **Do you have excessive bleeding with your period? (25,000 IU)** _____

7. **Do you have rough sandpaperlike skin on the backs of your arms? (10,000 IU)** _____
8. **Is your diet high in processed, canned, and cured meats, such as franks, salami, bologna, and sausages? (10,000 IU)** _____
9. **Are you exposed to air pollution or toxic chemicals? (10,000 IU)** _____
10. **Do you have a family history of cancer? (10,000 IU)** _____

   Basic Protection: 10,000 IU
   Maximum Dosage: 25,000 IU for 1 month, then 15,000 IU
   Your Dosage: _____

Vitamin B₁ (Thiamine)

Vitamin B$_1$ is necessary for carbohydrate metabolism. It helps maintain a healthy nervous system, stimulates growth and good muscle tone, and it has also been shown to stabilize the appetite.

The best sources of B$_1$ are wheat germ, blackstrap molasses, brewers' yeast, and bran. Whole-grain baked products are good for you because they contain generous amounts of B$_1$.

Vitamin B$_1$ is water-soluble and has no known toxicity level. You may notice that B$_1$ colors the urine a bright yellow, but the effect is harmless.

For each question that applies to you, add the appropriate amount of B$_1$. Vitamin B$_1$ is best taken in divided dosages three times a day.

1. **Is your diet high in white rice, white flour, white sugar, alcohol, and/or coffee? (50 mg.)** _____
2. **Do you have cracks or redness at the corners of your mouth or around your nose, or chronically chapped lips? (50 mg.)** _____
3. **Do you have problems healing cuts and wounds? (50 mg.)** _____

4. Have you been feeling depressed, irritable, and unable to concentrate? (50 mg.) _____

5. Have you been drinking more alcohol and eating a poor diet? (50 mg.) _____

6. Are you over sixty years of age? (50 mg.) _____

7. Has your tongue become deeply fissured or does it appear "pebbled"? (50 mg.) _____

   Basic Protection: 50 mg.
   Maximum Dosage: 100 mg.
   Your Dosage: _____

Vitamin B_2 (Riboflavin) Vitamin B_2 is necessary for carbohydrate, fat, and protein metabolism. It aids in the formation of antibodies and red blood cells, and helps maintain cell respiration. It also promotes good vision and helps keep skin, nails, and hair healthy.

Common sources of B_2 include organ meats, eggs, and milk, but because it's found in such minute amounts in those sources, it's difficult to get enough B_2 without taking a supplement.

Vitamin B_2 is water-soluble and has no known toxicity. However, large doses of B_2 (or any one of the other B vitamins, for that matter) may reduce the effectiveness of the other B vitamins.

For each question that applies to you, add the appropriate amount of vitamin B_2. You can take B_2 at one time during the day.

1. Do you have ulcerations or painful fissures at the corners of your mouth? (50 mg.) _____

2. Do you have scaly skin lesions around the nose, cheeks, chin, or ear lobes? (50 mg.) _____

3. Do you have constantly gritty or bloodshot eyes? (50 mg.) _____

4. Do you drink more than four alcoholic beverages per day? (50 mg.) _____

5. Do you have food idiosyncrasies or a habit of bad diet? (50 mg.) _____

6. Have you become sensitive to light? Do you suffer from eye strain? Do your eyes tear excessively? (50 mg.) _____

7. Have you been told that you are developing cataracts? (50 mg.) _____

8. Are you a physically active young woman? (50 mg.) _____

9. Have you been told that your thyroid function was sluggish or below normal? (50 mg.) _____

10. Have you been taking Elavil or Thorazine as medication? (50 mg.) _____

11. Are you taking birth control medication? (50 mg.) _____

12. Are you on a high-protein diet? (50 mg.) _____

    Basic Protection: 50 mg.

    Maximum Dosage: 100–300 mg.

    Your Dosage: _____

Vitamin B_3 (Niacin)

Vitamin B_3 is necessary for carbohydrate, fat, and protein metabolism. It helps maintain the health of your skin, tongue, digestive system, and nervous system, and it plays a role in the production of sex hormones. Vitamin B_3 also helps reduce cholesterol levels.

Vitamin B_3 is water-soluble and has no known toxicity, but it may cause a skin flush or itching in some people if they increase their dosage dramatically. The effect is harmless and usually disappears in thirty to sixty minutes. You can avoid the flush by taking B_3 in its slow-release form or by reducing the amount of B_3 you take.

For each question that applies to you, add the appropriate amount of B_3. To avoid flush and itching, increase the amount in 50-milligram increments. Vitamin B_3 is best taken in divided dosages three times daily.

1. Do you have elevated cholesterol? Do you have elevated triglycerides? (400 mg.) _____
2. Do you have osteoarthritis with impaired joint mobility? (250 mg., four times daily) _____
3. Do you have cracks or redness at the corners of your mouth and around your nose, or chronically chapped lips? (50 mg.) _____
4. Do you have a red-colored tongue that is heavily grooved or has become very smooth? (50 mg.) _____
5. Do you have ringing in your ears? (1,000 mg.) _____
6. Do you drink more than two alcoholic beverages per day? (50 mg.) _____
   Basic Protection: 50 mg.
   Maximum Dosage: 1,000 mg.
   Your Dosage: _____

Vitamin B_6

Vitamin B_6 is necessary for carbohydrate, fat, and protein metabolism. It is also instrumental in maintaining a normal balance of sodium and potassium in the body; this balance is essential for the normal functioning of the nervous, muscular, and skeletal systems. Vitamin B_6 also aids in the production of red blood cells and antibodies.

Meats and whole grains are the best sources of B_6.

Although vitamin B_6 is water-soluble, in dosages over 2,000 milligrams it may cause nerve disorders. An unsteady gait and numb feet are typical symptoms. Discontinuing the vitamin will eliminate these symptoms.

For each question that applies to you, add the appropriate amount of B_6 vitamin. B_6 is best taken in divided dosages three times a day at meals.

1. Do you suffer from the "Chinese restaurant syndrome," a response to MSG that includes headache? (50 mg.) _____

2. Do you suffer from premenstrual symptoms, particularly water retention? (200 mg., three times daily) _____

3. Are you taking birth control pills? (50 mg.) _____

4. Do you have low blood sugar or diabetes? (50 mg.) _____

5. Do you have carpal tunnel syndrome? Do you wake in the morning with numbness and tingling in your fingers? (200 mg., three times daily) _____

6. Do you have difficulty remembering your dreams? (50 mg.) _____

7. Do you suffer from kidney stones? (200 mg.) _____
   Basic Protection: 50 mg.
   Maximum Dosage: 600 mg.
   Your Dosage: _____

Vitamin B_{12}

Vitamin B_{12} is essential for normal formation of blood cells. It's necessary for carbohydrate, fat, and protein metabolism, and helps maintain a healthy nervous system.

The best sources of vitamin B_{12} include liver, kidneys, fish, red meats, and dairy products.

Vitamin B_{12} is water-soluble and has no known toxicity level. For each question that applies to you, add the appropriate amount of B_{12}. Vitamin B_{12} supplements are best taken at one time with meals.

1. Are you on a high-fiber diet? (1,000 mcg.) _____

2. Have you been excessively tired lately? Have you been under stress? (1,000 mcg.) _____

3. Do you suffer from recurrent canker sores? (1,000 mcg.) _____

4. Do you suffer from xanthelasma, or fatty deposits around the eyes? (1,000 mcg.) _____

5. Do you suffer from chronic bursitis of the shoulder? Do you have painful shoulders or

have you been told that you have calcium deposits in your shoulders? (1,000 mcg.) _____

6. Are you a strict vegetarian? (1,000 mcg.) _____
7. Are you taking high doses of folic acid? (1,000 mcg.) _____

    Basic Protection: 1,000 mcg.
    Maximum Dosage: 3,000 mcg.
    Your Dosage: _____

Pantothenic Acid

Pantothenic acid, part of the vitamin B complex, aids in the formation of some fats. It helps release energy from carbohydrates, fats, and protein, and aids in the utilization of some vitamins. It also improves the body's resistance to stress and helps maintain healthy nerves. There's some evidence that pantothenic acid can prevent premature aging as well as wrinkles.

The best sources of pantothenic acid include organ meats as well as brewers' yeast, whole-grain products, and egg yolks.

Pantothenic acid is water-soluble and has no known toxicity level. For each question that applies to you, add the appropriate amount of pantothenic acid. It is best taken in divided dosages, two to four times daily.

1. Do you suffer from rheumatoid arthritis? (250 mg., three times daily) _____
2. Are you prone to recurrent sore throats, colds, and viral infections? (200 mg.) _____
3. Do you suffer from ulcerative colitis or Crohn's disease? (200–1,000 mg.) _____
4. Do you feel stressed? (200 mg.) _____
5. Do you grind your teeth at night or feel excessive tension in your jaw? (200 mg.) _____

    Basic Protection: 50 mg.
    Maximum Dosage: 250–1,000 mg.
    Your Dosage: _____

Folic Acid

Folic acid is important in red-blood-cell formation. It aids in the metabolism of proteins and is necessary for growth and division of body cells. Folic acid is essential to your emotional and mental health.

Folic acid, if taken in doses over 1 milligram per day (1,000 micrograms), can mask the symptoms of pernicious anemia, which often results from a vitamin B_{12} deficiency. The extra folic acid can actually prevent the diagnosis of the disease before irreversible damage has occurred. Obviously it's important to confirm that you do not have a B_{12} deficiency before taking more than 800 micrograms per day of folic acid.

Nutritional surveys have shown that folic acid is frequently missing in our diets. The best sources of folic acid include liver, green leafy vegetables, and brewers' yeast.

Folic acid is water-soluble and has no known toxicity level, although, as mentioned above, an excessive intake can mask a B_{12} deficiency.

For each question that applies to you, add the appropriate amount of folic acid. Your dose may be taken all at one time with meals.

1. Are you taking birth control pills? (800 mcg.) _____
2. Have you been told that you have erosion of the cervix or cervical dysplasia? (1,600 mcg.) _____
3. Do you drink more than four alcoholic beverages per day? (800 mcg.) _____
4. Are you suffering from postpartum depression? Have you been feeling mildly depressed? (800 mcg.) _____

   Basic Protection: 400 mcg.
   Maximum Dosage: 2,000 mcg. (2 mg.)
   Your Dosage: _____

Vitamin C

Vitamin C helps heal wounds, scar tissue, and fractures. It maintains collagen and gives strength to blood vessels. It may provide resistance to infections. It aids in the absorption of iron. Vitamin C is important in the formation of epinephrine, one of the antistress hormones, because when the body is stressed, its store of vitamin C is quickly used up.

The most common sources of vitamin C include fresh fruits and vegetables, such as citrus fruits, strawberries, and tomatoes as well as green peppers, potatoes, and dark green vegetables.

Vitamin C is water-soluble and has no known toxicity level. Dr. Linus Pauling, Nobel Laureate Professor of Chemistry, recommends that most adults take between 250 and 10,000 milligrams (or 10 grams) daily. I've never seen toxicity symptoms with extremely large doses of vitamin C, although some patients report increased urination and/or increased bowel movements. Large doses of vitamin C should be avoided by people with a tendency to form kidney stones.

I don't think that there is any difference in effectiveness between "natural" and "synthetic" vitamin C. Most vitamin C is made from corn products. However, a noncorn-based vitamin C might be a better choice, as corn sometimes causes allergic reactions. Check the label to see if the C is derived from corn. If the label specifies "hypoallergenic," the vitamin C probably does not come from corn.

- For each question that applies to you, add the appropriate amount of C. Vitamin C is best taken in divided doses, two to four times daily.

1. Are you prone to frequent colds and other infections? (1,000–2,000 mg.) ——

2. Do you suffer from allergies? (1,000–2,000 mg.) ——

3. Do you suffer from irritated or infected gums? (1,000–2,000 mg.) _____
4. Do you smoke? (1,000 mg.) _____
5. Do you have a family history of cancer? (1,000 mg.) _____
6. Do you suffer from cervical dysplasia? (1,000 mg.) _____
7. Do you have a family history of heart disease? Do you have elevated cholesterol? Have you had a heart attack? (1,000 mg.) _____
8. Do you find that cuts and wounds are slow to heal? (1,000 mg.) _____
9. If you are a male with an infertility problem, has it been diagnosed as agglutination or clumping of sperm cells? (1,000 mg.) _____
10. Do you suffer from asthma? (1,000 mg.) _____
11. Are you exposed to highly polluted air or to smokers? (1,000 mg.) _____
12. Do your gums bleed easily when you brush your teeth? (1,000 mg.) _____
13. Are you taking iron supplements for iron-deficiency anemia? (500 mg.) _____

> Basic Protection: 1,000 mg.
> Maximum Dosage: 3,000 mg.
> Your Dosage: _____

Bioflavinoids

Bioflavinoids work in the body in conjunction with vitamin C. All their effects are not known, but they do help increase the strength of your capillaries and help protect your stores of vitamin C.

The most common sources of bioflavinoids include raw fruits and vegetables.

Bioflavinoids have no known toxicity level and are best taken with vitamin C. For each question that applies to you, add the appropriate amount of bioflavinoids.

1. Do you suffer from bleeding gums? (1,000 mg.) _____

2. Do you suffer from excessively heavy periods or bleeding between periods? (1,000 mg.) _____

3. Do you bruise easily? (1,000 mg.) _____

4. Do you have bleeding hemorrhoids? (1,000 mg.) _____

Basic Protection: 500 mg.
Maximum Dosage: 1,000 mg.
Your Dosage: _____

Vitamin D

Vitamin D improves the absorption and utilization of calcium and phosphorus required for the formation of bones. It maintains a stable nervous system and normal heart action.

Sunlight is the best natural source of vitamin D, but fish oils also contain it as well as egg yolks and fortified milk.

Vitamin D should be taken only when calcium and phosphorus requirements are being met, because otherwise no benefits will result.

Taken in excess of 1,000 IU over an extended period of time, vitamin D may be toxic for some people. For each question that applies to you, add the appropriate amount of D. Vitamin D may be taken at one time and is best taken with meals.

1. Do you have symptoms that may indicate calcium deficiency, such as recurrent nighttime leg cramps, heavy plaque around your teeth, a tendency toward kidney stone formation, osteoarthritic changes in the joints? (400 IU) _____

2. Do you live in northern climates where you are rarely exposed to sunlight? (400 IU) _____

3. Do you suffer from osteoporosis? (400 IU) _____
4. Are you pregnant or breast-feeding? (400 IU) _____

      Basic Protection: 400 IU
      Maximum Dosage: 800 IU
      Your Dosage: _____

Vitamin E

Vitamin E, an antioxidant, protects against the damage of free radicals in the body. These destructive molecules can cause everything from cancer to blood clots to premature aging. In addition, proper cellular respiration of the muscles, particularly the skeletal and cardiac muscles, is dependent on the presence of vitamin E.

The best natural sources of vitamin E include whole-grain cereals, wheat germ, vegetable oils, margarine, eggs, and green leafy vegetables.

Of the various forms of vitamin E, D-alpha tocopherol is the most potent and usable by the body. Look for this designation on the label when you buy E.

A fat-soluble vitamin, E is considered nontoxic except if given in large amounts to people with high blood pressure or chronic rheumatic heart disease. If you suffer from either of these conditions, don't take vitamin E unless supervised by a physician. It should not be taken with iron or birth control pills, as they neutralize the vitamin's activity. Take vitamin E at least six hours before or after either of these two substances. Don't take vitamin E if you are also taking anticoagulant drugs, such as Coumadin. If you take vitamin E and notice that you have prolonged bleeding from a cut or wound or if you develop unexplained bruises, I recommend discontinuing this supplement.

For each question that applies to you, add the appropriate amount of E. Vitamin E is best taken in divided dosages with meals.

1. **Are you exposed to air pollution or toxic chemicals? (400 IU)** _____
2. **Have you been told you have cystic breasts? (600 IU)** _____
3. **Do you get leg cramps after walking several hundred yards? (400 IU)** _____
4. **Do you have a family history of cancer? (800 IU)** _____
5. **Do you suffer from hot flashes or other menopausal symptoms? (800 IU)** _____
6. **Do you suffer from premenstrual syndrome? (800 IU)** _____
7. **Do you suffer from inflammation of the veins, phlebitis, or blood-clot formation? (400–800 IU)** _____
8. **Do you have a problem digesting fats? (400 IU)** _____

> Basic Protection: 400 IU
> Maximum Dosage: 1,200 IU
> Your Dosage: _____

Minerals

Calcium

Calcium, one of the major minerals, is essential for human life. It sustains the development and maintenance of your bones and teeth. It is also crucial for blood coagulation, muscle action, nerve function, heartbeat, the production of energy, and the maintenance of your immune system.

Lack of calcium in the bones, or osteoporosis, is recognized as one of the major health problems among the elderly, particularly women. Once women are past menopause, reduced estrogen makes it difficult for the bones to retain calcium. But it isn't enough merely to take calcium supplements, since only 20 or 30 percent of the calcium in these tablets is absorbed. The solution is exercise: It forces the calcium to interact with the bones and thus it is more readily absorbed. To maintain a healthy level of calcium in your bones, you should walk at least thirty minutes every day, or the equivalent in exercise.

The best sources of calcium include milk and other dairy products, eggs, sardines, green leafy vegetables, citrus fruits, and dried peas and beans.

Most people's diets are deficient in calcium, especially the low-fat diets that help prevent cardiovascular disease. Therefore calcium supplementation is recommended. I have experimented with taking a number of different calcium supplements at different times of day, and have found that ingesting calcium with meals seems to inhibit its absorption. I now take a liquid calcium preparation at bedtime, and it gives good results.

There is no known toxicity level for calcium, but people who suffer from kidney stones should check with their doctor before taking calcium supplements.

1. Are you over sixty years of age? (500 mg.) _____
2. Are you postmenopausal? (1,500 mg.) _____
3. Do you use antacids? (500 mg.) _____
4. Do you drink two or more alcoholic beverages per day? (500 mg.) _____
5. Do you have an intolerance to milk, or do you limit your intake of dairy products? (1,500 mg.) _____
6. Do you follow a high-protein or high-fiber diet? (500 mg.) _____
7. Have you been told that you have osteoporosis? (1,500–3,000 mg.) _____
8. Do you have trouble falling asleep? (1,500 mg. before bed) _____
9. Do you suffer from high blood pressure? (1,000 mg.) _____
10. Do you suffer from leg cramps at night? (1,500 mg.) _____

11. Do you have severe menstrual cramps?
    (1,500 mg.)   _____
12. Are you generally inactive and get no physi-
    cal exercise? (500 mg.)   _____
        Basic Protection: 1,000 mg.
        Maximum Dosage: 3,000 mg.
        Your Dosage: _____

Magnesium

Magnesium, a mineral essential for life, is necessary for every biological process. It is a catalyst in the utilization of carbohydrates, fats, and proteins as well as of certain minerals, including calcium, phosphorus, and perhaps potassium.

The best natural sources of magnesium include raw green leafy vegetables, almonds and cashew nuts, soybeans, and whole grains. Many people get inadequate amounts of magnesium from food. The typical individual receives barely the minimum RDA level of magnesium, which, as I've pointed out, is almost always insufficient.

There is evidence that suggests a balance between calcium and magnesium is particularly important, so I usually recommend taking four times as much calcium as magnesium.

1. Are you elderly? (200 mg.)   _____
2. Are you on a low-calorie diet? (200 mg.)   _____
3. Are you a diabetic? (200 mg.)   _____
4. Are you taking diuretics? (200 mg.)   _____
5. Do you drink more than one alcoholic
   beverage per day? (200 mg.)   _____
6. Are you pregnant? (200 mg.)   _____
7. Do you exercise regularly and strenuous-
   ly? (200 mg.)   _____
8. Do you have a family history of cardiovas-

cular disease or are you suffering from
cardiovascular disease? (200 mg.) _____

9. Do you have high blood pressure? (200
   mg.) _____
10. Do you have premenstrual syndrome? (200
    mg.) _____
11. Do you have kidney stones? (200 mg.) _____
12. Do you have recurrent bouts of diarrhea?
    (200 mg.) _____
13. Do you have ulcerative colitis or regional
    ileitis? (200 mg.) _____
14. Do you use laxatives frequently? (200 mg.) _____

   Basic Protection: 200 mg.
   Maximum Dosage: 400 mg.
   Your Dosage: _____

Chromium

Chromium, a trace mineral, stimulates enzymes in the
metabolism of energy—the processing of sugar in the
body—and also in the synthesis of fatty acids, cholesterol, and protein. It increases the effective use of insulin
by your body. For a complete discussion of chromium,
see page 92.

Brewers' yeast is a good source of chromium, as are
meat, cheese, cereals, and whole-grain breads.

Trivalent chromium is the form of chromium most
readily available to the body. There is no known toxicity
level for chromium. For each question that applies to
you, add the appropriate amount of chromium. Chromium is best taken before meals in divided dosages.

1. Do you have periods during the day when
   you feel tired, irritable, fatigued, moody,
   and you cannot concentrate? (100 mcg.) _____
2. Are you over sixty years of age? (150 mcg.) _____
3. Are you pregnant? (150 mcg.) _____

4. Do you have a high consumption of refined foods (such as white sugar, desserts, cookies, candy, ice cream, etc.)? (300 mcg.) _____
5. Do you exercise strenuously? (150 mcg.) _____
6. Do you have cardiovascular disease? (150 mcg.) _____
7. Do you have hypoglycemia? (300 mcg.) _____
8. Do you have diabetes? (300 mcg.) _____
    Basic Protection: 200 mcg.
    Maximum Dosage: 600 mcg.
    Your Dosage: _____

Selenium

Selenium has received a great deal of attention as one of the "super-nutrients." It is said to inhibit the major effects of aging and to reduce the incidence of many diseases, i.e., cancer and heart disease. Whether or not these claims are true, we do know that selenium is an antioxidant and appears to preserve the elasticity of tissues. It also enhances the action of vitamin E. I believe that selenium is an important antistress nutrient.

The best natural sources of selenium include broccoli, mushrooms, cabbage, celery, cucumbers, onions, radishes, brewers' yeast, whole grains, fish, and organ meats.

For each question that applies to you, add the appropriate amount of selenium. Selenium is best taken in divided dosages.

1. Do you have a family history of cancer? (50 mcg.) _____
2. Do you have frequent sore throats or colds? (50 mcg.) _____
3. Do you have a family history of heart disease? (50 mcg.) _____
4. Do you have angina (chest pains)? (50 mcg.) _____

5. Are you exposed to air pollution or toxic chemicals? (50 mcg.) _____
6. Do you drink more than one alcoholic drink per day? (50 mcg.) _____
7. Do you smoke cigarettes or are you exposed to cigarette smoke? (50 mcg.) _____
8. Do you eat a diet high in fat? (50 mcg.) _____
   Basic Protection: 50–100 mg.
   Maximum Dosage: 200 mg.
   Your Dosage: _____

Zinc

Zinc is an important mineral that aids the immune system in its efforts to prevent disease. It also helps in digestion and the metabolism of phosphorus, and aids the healing process. There is increasing evidence that many people are deficient in their intake of zinc.

The best natural sources of zinc include meat, liver, poultry, fish, dairy products, and whole grains.

There doesn't seem to be a toxicity level to zinc intake, although people who take megadoses could suffer side effects.

For each following question that applies to you, add the appropriate amount of zinc. As zinc is one of the most common minerals that may cause gastric upset, it is best to take it in divided dosages with food. Since a high-fiber diet can diminish the amount of zinc you are able to absorb, it is probably best to take it at meals other than breakfast.

1. Do you get frequent colds and sore throats? (50 mg.) _____
2. Do you have difficulty with your sense of smell or taste? (100 mg.) _____
3. Do you find that cuts and wounds are slow to heal? (50 mg.) _____

4. Do you suffer from gastric ulcers? (50 mg.)____

5. Do you have a problem with potency and sex drive? (100–200 mg.) ____

6. Do you have a prostate problem? (100–200 mg.) ____

7. Do you have diabetes or a carbohydrate imbalance such as hypoglycemia? (100 mg.) ____

8. Are you taking cortisone drugs? (50 mg.) ____

9. Do you suffer from acne? (100 mg.) ____

10. Do you get recurrent boils? (100 mg.) ____

11. Do you have body odor that defies control? (100 mg.) ____

12. Do you suffer from rheumatoid arthritis? (50 mg.) ____

13. Have you been told that you are infertile because of a low sperm count? (100–200 mg.) ____

14. Are you a heavy smoker? (50 mg.) ____

15. Do you suffer from osteoarthritis? (50 mg., four times daily) ____

   Basic Protection: 50 mg.
   Maximum Dosage: 200 mg.
   Your Dosage: _____

Copper

Copper is one of the trace minerals that has recently been recognized as crucial to human metabolism. It is necessary in the formation of red blood cells, important in the effective functioning of the nervous system, and is part of many enzymes. It works with vitamin C to form elastin, the protein responsible for the elasticity of the lungs, blood vessels, and skin. There is some evidence that copper may protect against cancer and cardiovascular disease, and that it is of some help in relieving arthritis.

The best food sources of copper include oysters, liver,

kidneys, dried beans, corn-oil margarine, whole-grain products, and green leafy vegetables. Drinking water may also be a source of this mineral, which leaches from copper piping.

Because there is still a great deal of research to be done on copper, I simply recommend that you take a basic protection dosage. As copper complements zinc in its function in the body, it's important that you take ten times as much zinc as copper. Whatever you figured as your dosage of zinc, divide it by ten to get your copper dosage.

> **Basic Protection: 2 mg.**
> **Your Dosage:** _____

Iron

Iron is recognized now as a trace mineral essential for human life. It is necessary for blood formation. It also aids in the metabolism of protein and promotes growth.

The best natural sources of iron include liver, kidneys, red meats, oysters, egg yolks, green leafy vegetables, dried fruits, potatoes, and enriched and whole-grain cereals.

Iron supplements may cause intestinal cramping, diarrhea, or constipation, and may color the stool a very dark brown or black. If you develop these symptoms, take the supplement once or twice a week rather than daily. If they persist, consult your physician concerning changing the type of iron.

Excessive intake of iron may be toxic, although such cases are very rare. For each question that applies to you, add the appropriate amount of iron. It is best taken between meals, and since vitamin C helps in its absorption while calcium diminishes its effectiveness, it is preferable to take iron with a glass of orange juice than with a glass of milk.

1. Do you avoid red meat? (60 mg.) _____
2. Have you been told that you are anemic because of blood loss from heavy periods, overuse of aspirin, hiatus hernia, peptic ulcers, colitis, diverticular disease, or hemorrhoids? (60 mg.) _____
3. Do you have lowered resistance to infection? Do you get frequent colds and sore throats? (60 mg.) _____
4. Do you engage in endurance sports? Have you been especially tired lately after working out? (60 mg.) _____
5. Are you pregnant? (60 mg.) _____
    Basic Protection: 60 mg.
    Maximum Dosage: 120 mg.
    Your Dosage: _____

Iodine

Iodine, a trace mineral, is present in very small quantities in your body. It controls the speed of your metabolism by affecting the production of the thyroid hormone thyroxine. Iodine is crucial to the effective functioning of your heart, your immune system, and your body's ability to synthesize protein.

Good sources of natural iodine include all types of seafoods, mushrooms, seaweed products, iodized salt, and sea salt.

People on an extremely salt-limited diet might be directed to take one or two kelp tablets (15 micrograms) to add some iodine. However, I believe the iodine found in our basic protection multiple-vitamin supplement is sufficient.

Natural vs. Synthetic Vitamins

In general, a vitamin is a vitamin is a vitamin. Natural and synthetic versions of the same substance are chemically identical. It has been argued that natural vitamins contain some still unidentified nutrients that may be beneficial, but I do not recommend natural vitamins over synthetic vitamins, which are usually less expensive.

Adverse Reactions to Vitamins?

Although there may be isolated medical reports of vitamin and mineral toxicity from supplementation in high dosages, I have never seen a toxic reaction, although many patients have had allergic or hypersensitivity reactions. These may include headaches, nausea, fatigue, palpitations, or loose bowel movements. These reactions will occur within one or two days of beginning the supplements and will cease when they are discontinued. If a reaction occurs, discontinue all supplements and reintroduce them one at a time at four-day intervals until a reaction signals the problem supplement. I do not think that these are toxic reactions, but rather a hypersensitivity reaction to the binders, fillers, coatings, or the product from which the supplement is derived.

For example, most vitamin C is derived from corn, and many patients are sensitive to corn products and thus will not be able to take this type of vitamin C. Additionally, many supplements are prepared in a yeast base; many of my patients are sensitive to yeast and react to a multitude of supplements. Therefore, I always recommend hypoallergenic supplements; that is, they contain no corn, wheat, lactose, yeast, binders, fillers, chemicals, or other allergenic materials.

After many trials, I have found that the best-tolerated

and best-absorbed supplements are the pure vitamin or mineral powders in gelatin capsules. To ensure maximum tolerance and absorption, these products contain no dilutants, preservatives, binders, or excipients.

Week Five: Alcohol

Do you drink regularly—say, wine with dinner or a few beers in the evening—but feel certain that your drinking is completely under control because you're rarely, if ever, inebriated? If so, this week of the Makeover will be an important one for you. In the course of my practice, I've discovered that many people who are certainly not alcoholics have a special kind of drinking problem. Many of them are never inebriated, and they never let alcohol interfere with their work or their personal lives, but they suffer from the consequences of their drinking nonetheless. If you've made alcohol a part of your daily life and you are not aware of the harm it is doing to your current and future health, then this week of the Makeover will be a big step forward on your road to increased energy, vitality, and optimum health.

This Week's Goal

The nation seems to be divided into three groups of alcohol consumers, and about one third of them don't drink at all or rarely have a drink, another third have up to three drinks each week, and the final third have four or more drinks each week. If you don't drink or do so rarely, then you can skip the fifth week of the Makeover and move ahead to the exercise week. If you have up to three drinks weekly, you'll find this week is easy, but I still suggest that you complete it in sequence. If you drink four or more drinks weekly, then this will be an important week for you because you may discover that alcohol has become a psychological addiction. You probably won't find this week difficult, but it is very important from physical and psychological standpoints. Many of my patients tell me that the fifth week is a real turning point because it encourages them to scrutinize a habit that they feel is essential to their business and personal lives, and discover a great sense of satisfaction in coming to terms with it in a positive way.

Alcohol is a fact of life for Americans. Even though alcohol is a drug that has ruined countless lives, it is advertised as a sophisticated, pleasurable, adult "treat." It's part and parcel of a relaxing evening with friends, it's the core of the cocktail party, it's an icebreaker at any gathering, it's even donated by airlines to compensate for a flight delay. This benign acceptance of alcohol denies its dangerous properties and encourages you to make it a regular part of your life. If you drink now and want to continue to drink in the future—which describes the desire of most of my patients—I don't think you need banish alcohol from your life forever. But you do need to change your attitude toward alcohol and change the role it plays in your life. If you want to enjoy optimum health, you can't afford to let alcohol become a habit.

No, you do not have to give up alcohol forever. As you might imagine, this is the first question many of my patients ask me. But you do have to give it up completely for one week—Week Five—of the Makeover. There are two reasons for this limited abstention: One is to prove that you can do it and the other is to demonstrate to yourself how you feel when you haven't had a drink in a week. After this week you'll be able to drink, but on a limited basis, for the rest of the Makeover. Your first week without alcohol will give you a feeling of self-mastery that will extend into the remaining three weeks of the Makeover and will help you stick to your newly limited alcohol consumption. You may be surprised to find that those one or two drinks you have been accustomed to having every night are having a much bigger effect on the way you feel every day than you imagined.

Dean Martin has joked that he feels sorry for people who don't drink because when they wake up in the morning, that's as good as they're going to feel all day. If you drink regularly, the morning may well be the lowest point of your day because you're always suffering from a slight hangover. But when you stop drinking, even for a week, and wake up feeling fresh and alert, this will give you a new perspective on the role alcohol plays in your life.

Alcoholics and the Makeover

This week of the Makeover is not geared to alcoholics. It is not a program for people who are physically addicted to alcohol. Though we have talked about physical addictions like caffeine and sugar and, I hope, have conquered them, alcoholism is a far more serious disease. Confirmed alcoholics—about seventeen million Americans—need more help than a week of the Makeover can provide. It's almost impossible to combat alcoholism without outside assistance. If you have a physical addiction to alcohol, I suggest you get in touch with Alcoholics Anonymous, P.O. Box 459, Grand Central Station, New York, NY 10017. They'll be able to give you the address of your local Alcoholics Anonymous chapter.

Most people know if their drinking is a serious problem, or at least they suspect it. The following symptoms, from Dr. Morris Chafetz, former director of the National Institute on Alcohol Abuse and Alcoholism, are indications of a drinking problem:

- Anyone who has been drunk four times a year
- Anyone who drinks in order to work
- Anyone who goes to work intoxicated
- Anyone who is intoxicated and drives a car
- Anyone who sustains bodily injury requiring medical attention as the consequence of drinking
- Anyone who comes in conflict with legal authority as a consequence of drinking
- Anyone who, under the influence of alcohol, does something he would not otherwise do.

If you have any of these symptoms, I urge you to get professional help to cope with your drinking.

The New Problem Drinker

A few of my patients are recovered alcoholics and some don't drink at all, but most are what I consider the new "problem" drinkers. These are not people who have a serious problem with alcohol, but rather people for whom drinking has become a part of their daily routine. They no longer think about whether they want to have a drink, and many acknowledge that they don't even take a great deal of pleasure in drinking. At routine times of the day or evening they simply have a drink. Most of these individuals are convinced that the pressures of their work or lifestyle demand that they drink. Either they must have a drink because their job entails entertaining, or they must have one because they need it to relax at the end of the day, or they must have wine with dinner because they can't imagine enjoying a meal without wine.

Greg H., who works with computer graphics and animation, was typical of many of my patients in his relationship to alcohol. Greg first came to see me because he suffered from recurring colds. It seemed that as soon as he recovered from one cold, he began to develop another. His first appointment was in the early spring and he told me he had had about seven colds that winter. When I asked Greg if he drank, he said, "No." But then he quickly added, "Well, I guess just the normal amount." The "normal amount" was from one half to three quarters of a bottle of wine a night. Greg and his wife both worked long hours and dinner was a bit of a ceremony for them—an occasion to unwind from the day and catch up with each other. Years ago they began to have a glass of wine with dinner. Over time, that glass turned into a half-bottle each. Every once in a while they would open a second bottle and have another glass or two.

Greg and his wife felt they should be drinking less. Now and again, they would skip the nightly bottle, but they would somehow feel deprived and even a bit silly. They certainly didn't have a drinking problem, and they took so much pleasure from their evening wine that they couldn't convince themselves to give it up even for one night.

This kind of habitual drinking is a good example of what I consider the new "problem" drinking. Most people who drink this way are not going to become alcoholics, though, of course, some will. But they've made alcohol such an integral part of their lives that they've become psychological addicts. They suspect they may be drinking too much, but they don't realize what effect it's having on their health and they can't find any reason to give it up.

The goal of the Makeover is to break the pattern of the new "problem" drinker. This week of the Makeover is geared to breaking an essentially psychological dependence on alcohol. For those who find it particularly difficult to stop drinking, there is a supplement that should help them. But for most of you, understanding when and why you drink and how alcohol is affecting your health in the long and short terms is enough to get you through this week.

Taking Stock

When I asked Greg how much he drank and he answered "The normal amount," he couldn't have known how typical his response was. Most people think that whatever they drink is the normal amount. But in fact what I usually find is that many people not only don't know what an average amount of alcohol is, they don't even really know how much they drink themselves. Greg told me he had a half-bottle of wine most nights, so he was an exception to this rule. Many people say they have "a few glasses of wine" or a "couple of drinks," but the difference between the size of some wineglasses can be measured in many ounces, and we all know that certain restaurants and hosts are known for their generous pourings.

A drink usually means 0.5 ounces of absolute alcohol. From a practical standpoint, this means the drink could be one jigger (1½ ounces) of 80-proof distilled spirits, 1 ounce of 110-proof distilled spirits; one 12-ounce glass of beer; one 8-ounce glass of stout; one 5-ounce glass of French wine; one 4-ounce glass of American wine; 3 ounces of sherry.

Before you begin Week Five, it's helpful to know exactly how much you drink. Assess how much you drank last week. Try to remember every meal, party, or event where liquor was served and estimate how much you consumed. If you drink at home, take a minute to measure your glasses and how much alcohol is in each type of drink you make. If you drink at restaurants or parties, estimate how much alcohol was in each drink you had. The point of this exercise is to make you aware of how much you actually drink. If you drink in connection with business, you may be surprised to find that you're consuming far more than you had thought.

Knowing the amount of alcohol you consume is not the whole story. Liquor affects everyone differently and at a different rate of speed. If you are a slight woman, you may be adversely affected by two drinks, while a 250-pound man might barely react to the same amount. Moreover, if you drink on an empty stomach, you are affected more quickly. And finally, your body chemistry—the biochemical individuality we discussed in the vitamin-mineral week—determines to some degree the rate at which your body metabolizes alcohol. Some people have little tolerance for alcohol and can be adversely affected by just a few drinks, while other people seem to be able to tolerate large amounts of alcohol without behavioral changes.

Are You a New "Problem" Drinker?

I've found that for purposes of the Makeover, the emotional circumstances in which you drink are even more important than the amount. Mary M., a fundraiser for a national organization, illustrates this point. Mary told me that when she first came to New York, two, or sometimes three, nights a week would find her in one of the singles bars that line Third Avenue. Two or three times a month she would wake in the morning with a real hangover. Every time it happened, she would vow to drink less, and for a few weeks would hold to her resolution. She was very aware of the situations in which she drank and the consequences of her drinking.

After a few years Mary married. She and her husband

fell into the habit of having a drink as they prepared dinner together; they would have wine with dinner and perhaps a cordial at the end of the evening. This pattern built up gradually until the amount of liquor they consumed each night became routine. Mary said that, while she actually drank much less in her single days, she was far more aware of her drinking. But in the settled, companionable drinking with her husband, she had lost track of the fact that she was consuming a great deal of alcohol every night. She didn't notice its effects in the morning because there was no appreciable difference in how she felt from one day to the next. When in the course of her Makeover Mary broke the pattern of her drinking—as did her husband—she was surprised to discover how different she felt in the morning when she hadn't had a drink the night before.

Focus on the occasions that prompt you to drink:

- Is your drinking more a habit than a pleasure?
- Are there certain times each day when you have a drink without thinking about it?
- Do you drink the same amount nearly every day?
- Are you oblivious to how you feel the morning after drinking?
- Has your alcohol consumption increased steadily over a period of time to its present level?

If you answer yes to most of these questions, you may fall into my category of the new "problem" drinker, and it's time you broke the pattern.

"The French Do It . . ."

European habits have become the most gleefully embraced rationale of the new "problem" drinkers. They reason that because the French or the Italians or the

Greeks drink a half or a whole bottle, or one and half bottles of wine each day, it's appropriate and even sophisticated to do the same. I have no statistics to demonstrate that the French or any other European group drinks more regularly than Americans and, if they do, what effect it has on their health. Perhaps the stereotypical French obsession with the health of the liver is a legitimate concern about the damage excessive drinking is doing to it.

I mention the "European excuse" here because I've noticed how easy it is to ignore or excuse an increasing alcohol consumption. Most of us are well aware of the dangers of drinking and driving. The tragic results of that combination are in the newspapers every morning. Most of us feel that if we drink for business or relaxation, and we do it in moderate if regular amounts, and we don't drive in connection with our drinking, then we're being sensible about alcohol. What we ignore is the fact that if we drink regularly, we are running a significant health risk, not only because of the direct effect of alcohol on our bodies, particularly on our livers and gastrointestinal systems, but because its side effects can impair nutrition, and blood-sugar level.

The Two Faces of Alcohol

Alcohol is a food and a drug. Unfortunately, in both forms it has severe drawbacks that can be readily summarized: As a food—a carbohydrate—alcohol acts almost as an antinutrient because it increases your need for other nutrients while contributing virtually nothing of any nutritional value of its own. As a drug, alcohol's arguable benefit—its sedative value—is diminished because of the toxic effects it has on the brain, heart, liver, and gastrointestinal tract. The ready availability of alcohol exacerbates its drawbacks as both food and drug.

As a drug, alcohol is the most abused substance in this country. It is readily available, and its abuse is encouraged by advertising. We spend more than $20 billion each year on alcohol, and, despite its obvious dangers, it is a major source of revenue for our government: Tax revenues from the sale of alcohol are exceeded only by personal and corporate taxes. I suppose this is the only advantage of alcohol, though a dubious one, as it discourages concerted efforts by the government to fight the use of a drug that contributes to more than 100,000 deaths and $120 billion in economic losses yearly. I think one of the biggest failures of government and the health professions is the focus on drunk driving as the most serious side effect of drinking. This approach implies that as long as you don't drive, you can drink as much as you want. It ignores the irrefutable links between drinking and serious health problems.

Moderate Drinking: A Delicate Balance

Like sugar and caffeine, alcohol, in moderation, is considered by most people to be a benign substance. While I think that an occasional drink creates no problem for the healthy individual, I've found in creating the Makeover for my patients that moderate drinking is difficult to achieve and that anything short of moderate drinking can affect health directly as well as indirectly by reinforcing other bad habits.

Very few of my patients are true "moderate" drinkers. Most either drink very little or are habitual drinkers—the new "problem" drinkers whom I described above. Most of these people are mildly concerned about their drinking but not moved to do something about it. If you are a new "problem" drinker, you should know that you are living in a danger zone. Alcohol is a drug that encourages tolerance and this is the dangerous risk you're taking. When you first had a sip of liquor as a child or young adult, you felt it immediately and strongly. Over a period of time, as you consume more alcohol, it takes ever greater quantities for you to feel the same effects. Regular drinking regularly increases your tolerance.

Many of my patients find that, while they may have started out having a glass of wine with dinner, over time they have graduated to a half-bottle or more. If the only problem with drinking was just getting drunk—and these patients kept drinking more and were not getting drunk—such tolerance would be nothing to worry about. But increased tolerance—inevitable with regular drinking—is encouraging the drinker to consume more and more alcohol, a toxic substance that affects health more and more as consumption escalates. Of course, over time it becomes a case of diminishing returns: It takes more alcohol to feel any good effect, and that brief good effect takes an increasing toll on the body.

The regular drinker runs other risks: As his tolerance grows, a regular drinker will feel sober sooner than a true moderate drinker, even though his blood-alcohol level is higher. Feeling sober, he drives, conducts business, and otherwise performs tasks, such as operating machines that put him at risk of injury or even death. His abilities are impaired, but he feels as if he's sober.

Because of this tolerance, moderate drinking is difficult to achieve and begins seriously to affect the drinker's health as a result of the poison being introduced regularly to the system. But there is another risk. The moderate drinker is always in danger of becoming a problem drinker. Studies have shown that one out of every ten regular drinkers is likely to become a problem drinker or an alcoholic. The risk seems to be even higher for women because their bodies are more sensitive to the effects of alcohol. You don't become an alcoholic from having a few drinks—it takes time. In fact, the greater your tolerance to alcohol, the greater your potential for becoming an alcoholic. Men or women who can drink as if they had a hollow leg are likely to drink to excess because their bodies are not warning them of the toxicity of liquor. On the other hand, someone who passes out or feels nauseated after a few drinks is unlikely to continue to drink and build up a tolerance to, then a dependence on, alcohol.

Alcohol in Action

Alcohol moves with enormous speed through your body and affects every single tissue and organ. Alcohol enters and leaves the stomach quickly and is taken up by the small intestine. It is absorbed by the bloodstream in sixty to ninety seconds, and moves quickly to the liver, where most of it is metabolized.

It doesn't take much alcohol to affect the body dramatically. Just a few ounces will disorganize body tissues and cause water to migrate from within the cells to the spaces between them. Alcohol quickly affects the brain by interfering with the cells that protect the brain's capillaries from poison.

First, alcohol depresses your higher brain functions controlling vision, hearing, feeling, speech, thinking, attention span, and movement. Then alcohol begins to depress or slow your lower brain centers which control such vital functions as breathing, heart rate, and sleep.

Once alcohol enters your system a variety of physical changes occur that have short- and long-term effects on your health. Alcohol damages the following:

• THE BRAIN AND NERVOUS SYSTEM: You're familiar with those, most obvious, effects of alcohol: the slurred speech, aggressiveness, poor judgment, and increased risk of accidents. The increased risk of accidents is a very serious problem: The National Institute on Alcohol Abuse and Alcoholism claims that one out of every ten highway fatalities in the United States involves drinking. Thirty-five to 64 percent of drivers involved in fatal accidents were drinking, as are half of those who die in falls, 68 percent of those who drown, and 50 percent of those who die in fires. A single drink can impair your ability to recognize familiar objects in motion, tell one color from another, and recover from the glare of an oncoming headlight for a duration of *five to six hours*. In fact, it can take someone who's been drinking up to forty seconds to recover from the glare of approaching headlights, while a sober person will recover in half that time. It's easy to see why drinking makes you so vulnerable to accidents.

In addition, alcohol destroys brain cells, which, unlike the blood cells it also destroys, are irreplaceable. In a Danish study, when male alcoholics with an average age of thirty were tested for liver damage, only 19 percent had evidence of such damage, but 59 percent were discovered to be "intellectually impaired." After a period of only ten years of drinking, they had irreversibly damaged their brains.

There is no question that drinking impairs memory. It seems to do this by interfering with the brain cells' ability to build proteins, which are the basis of memory. Alcohol therefore damages your capacity for learning new things and your ability to remember what has happened in the past. Some researchers have even speculated that drinking is also an unrecognized cause of presenile dementia.

• SEXUAL PERFORMANCE: Many people think of alcohol as a substance that enhances sexuality because it dissolves inhibitions. But while that aspect of alcohol consumption may be true, its ultimate effect impairs follow-through. Even moderate amounts of alcohol impair a man's ability to achieve and maintain an erection. The result is temporary impotence—hardly a sexual enhancement. Men who drink excessively can also find that over a period of time the level of the male hormone testosterone is lowered and their bodies can become feminized with enlarged breasts.

• DRUG METABOLISM: Many people are familiar with the deadly relationship between drinking and tranquilizers. It's less well known that alcohol has an effect on many other kinds of drugs. In some cases alcohol impairs the drug, in others it increases its effect. Either situation can be especially dangerous because either can occur after a single drink. For example, antihistamines can amplify the alcohol's effect on the brain so that performance skills are even more severely impaired. Some of the drugs that alcohol interacts with include barbiturates, tranquilizers, anesthetics, morphine, antidepressant drugs, anticonvulsants, anticoagulants, antibiotics, and antihypertensives. In 1979 alcohol used in conjunction with other drugs was reported to be the most frequent cause of drug-related medical crises in the United States.

• THE GASTROINTESTINAL SYSTEM: Alcohol consumption leads to gastric irritation and eventually to a loss of part of the lining of the intestines. This loss impairs the absorption of lactose (the sugar found in milk), and ultimately results in an intolerance to milk and other dairy products. The damaged intestine is also less able to absorb certain nutrients, including thiamine and folic acid. A thiamine deficiency will affect the body's ability to metabolize carbohydrates; too little folic acid will lead to anemia and an inability to replace worn-out body tissues.

• THE LIVER: As the liver must do most of the work of metabolizing alcohol, it can suffer the most from the effects of these efforts. If you have more than three drinks each day, your liver will begin to accumulate fats. If you stop drinking, these fats will dissipate and your liver will recover. But if you continue to drink, you increase the risk of contracting alcoholic hepatitis—the inflammation and destruction of liver cells. Fifteen percent of those who drink heavily develop cirrhosis of the liver, irreversible scarring, and destruction of liver tissue.

• CANCER: People who drink regularly increase their risk of developing cancer. The link between drinking and cancer is not yet clear, but some of the proposed connections include the suppression of the immune system by alcohol, the effects of malnutrition related to drinking, the effects of repeated tissue contact with alcohol itself, or perhaps the carcinogenic substances found in alcoholic drinks. The cancers that have been linked to drinking include those of the liver, mouth, esophagus, pancreas, intestine, prostate, and lung.

Alcohol's Secret Stress

All the health hazards of alcohol mentioned above are well researched and documented. Unfortunately, many people, particularly the new "problem" drinkers, find it relatively easy to dismiss them. They don't really believe that they drink enough to impair the brain or liver, and they think that pollution or food additives are just as likely to cause cancer. But these people are ignoring one of the most subtle and damaging effects of alcohol: how it influences your ability to handle stress and how this reinforces your other bad health habits.

As I discussed earlier, stress is more than dealing with an angry boss. Your body can create its own biochemical stress as a result of foods you eat or don't eat, or simply as an amplification of its normal reaction to an outside stress. Alcohol, in addition to other effects on the body, also acts as a stress. It has recently been discovered that when alcohol enters the blood, it stimulates an increased production of the stress hormone norepinephrine. We have learned that this hormone has an immediate and dramatic effect on the body as it mobilizes all your resources to fight stress. The fact that alcohol stimulates norepinephrine production suggests that regular drinking is taking its toll on your body's ability to cope with other stressful areas of your life.

Alcohol and Blood Sugar

There is also a connection between alcohol and blood sugar that reinforces your bad habits. Alcohol is the most rapidly absorbed carbohydrate. It enters your system immediately and can create the same problems that a sudden overload of sugar does. If you have any problem with your blood sugar, as many of my patients do, you may find yourself predisposed to drinking. Because of stress or a poor diet or irregular meals, you may discover that at certain times of the day you're dying for an energy lift because your blood sugar is low. Your body has learned that alcohol will provide that lift. So, perhaps at lunch or before dinner you crave a drink. The drink makes your blood sugar soar and then, as we've learned, crash. The crash not only makes you feel tired and irritable and moody, it also makes you crave another high. This syndrome can encourage you to develop the bad habits of smoking, drinking, caffeine consumption, and eating sweets, all of which will temporarily raise your blood-sugar level.

You can see why at this stage in the Makeover, when you've given up caffeine and sugar and improved your nutrition and begun taking vitamin and mineral supplements, that you are better able to deal with the effects of drinking and to change your life pattern. You've loosened many of the ties to alcohol you may have had. But if you continue to drink habitually, it will be increasingly difficult to stick to your new good habits because alcohol will actually weaken your physiological resolve.

Alcohol's Most Ignored Danger

In the previous two weeks when we worked on nutrition and vitamins and mineral supplements we've seen how good nutrition is really the cornerstone of good health; and, indeed, suboptimum nutrition is responsible for a host of diseases as well as the vague symptoms we're trying to abolish. Alcohol is one of the most potent destroyers of good nutrition—and in my mind, that is one of its most serious side effects. By impairing good nutrition, alcohol creates immediate symptoms as well as encourages the development of chronic disease.

There are a number of ways in which alcohol encourages nutritional deficiency. For one thing, it diminishes appetite. While at first this might seem appealing if you're overweight, in fact, alcohol seems to encourage the regular drinker to gain. Many of my patients have experienced this syndrome. They go to a cocktail party after work and have a few drinks. By the time they have consumed several cocktails, they have little appetite, so they eat a small, and often eccentric, dinner—a few crudités or handfuls of corn chips. But the next morning, their blood sugar is extremely low, they're suffering from the effects of the alcohol, and they're ravenous. They eat enough the next day to more than make up for the calories they missed the evening before.

Even if you eat properly when you drink, you still run the risk of nutritional deficiency, because alcohol alters the function of all the gastrointestinal tract organs. It interferes with the digestion and absorption of nutrients and vitamins. In fact, it has been suggested that drinking is the most common cause of vitamin and trace-element deficiency in adults in the United States.

Alcohol also interferes with optimum nutrition because it provides nothing but empty calories. Alcohol has a high number of calories per ounce compared with other beverages, and many drinkers gain weight just by virtue of those excess calories. In fact, some people consume more calories in beer each day than they do in food. Obviously, over a period of time this can cause severe nutritional deficiency. Also the obesity that can result from drinking puts the drinker at risk for heart disease and cardiovascular disease.

As we have learned from the nutrition and vitamin-mineral weeks of the Makeover, just a marginal nutritional deficiency can cause both short- and long-term health problems. If you drink, you're making it even harder for your body to achieve optimum health.

Beginning Your Alcohol-Free Week

Because your addiction to alcohol is more psychological than physiological, planning for this week is a simple matter of understanding and anticipating the situations in which you may want to have a drink. You don't have to go shopping, but if it is your habit to have wine every night with dinner, then you could buy some seltzer to substitute for the wine. You do have to anticipate all the circumstances in which you would ordinarily drink, and you must plan ahead how to handle those situations. If you wait until someone is handing you a drink, you'll be forced to make a decision on the spot and risk having "just that one" because it's easier than dealing with refusal.

1. *Enlist the Help of Your Friends and Family.* If you usually have a drink after work with your spouse, try to convince him or her to help you by giving up the habit for at least this week. Make it a challenge for both of you. If your spouse resists, at least ask him or her to respect your decision and not pressure you to join in drinking.

2. *Learn to Say No.* This can be very difficult to do. If you regularly drink with others and face the possibility of

doing so this week, I suggest you prepare in advance how you're going to say no. Fortunately, today more people are conscious of their health, so a decision not to drink will usually be accepted without question. But if you have friends or business associates who pressure you to join them in a cocktail or wine with a meal, you must be prepared. One of my patients told me that he found the best response was to inform everyone he was on medication that wouldn't mix with alcohol. He only uses that as a last resort because in most cases people respect his refusal of a drink.

Another patient told me that she was very nervous about not drinking at lunch. She works in advertising and entertains clients almost every day. Though she usually just has one drink, some of her business contacts have as many as four. She felt that they would feel uncomfortable if she didn't drink at all. As it turned out, she had no difficulty handling the situation. She simply told them that she was on the Medical Makeover, and she described the program. Many of her lunch guests were interested to learn about the Makeover, and all seemed perfectly comfortable with her decision not to drink. One person even told her that he was relieved she wasn't drinking; he didn't really like to drink at lunch, but did it because it seemed unfriendly not to.

3. *Find Substitutes*. This isn't difficult to do. Plain seltzer with a lemon or lime wedge is the perfect drink to sip at a party. No one can tell you're not drinking something more potent. An orange or apple spritzer can make a good before-meal drink. Just mix orange or apple juice half and half with seltzer. If you entertain frequently at lunch and often go to the same restaurant, you can do what one of my patients did: Tell the waiter in advance that you just want a seltzer (or some other substitute) instead of a drink when cocktails are ordered. When everyone else orders drinks, you can just order "the usual."

4. *Find Substitute Routines*. Many people rely on alcohol to help them relax at the end of the day. In small amounts alcohol can be an effective relaxant, but, as we know, the problems for the habitual drinker are developing a tolerance and drinking increasing amounts. Therefore, you should never drink in order to unwind. Instead, do something else to relax, and make it a new habit. For example, one of my patients used to have a drink with her husband the minute they both got home from work. It was their time to catch up with each other, review the events of the day, and plan their evening. She couldn't imagine doing without that special time. When she came to the fifth week of the Makeover, she decided that the only solution would be to find another habit to substitute for the evening drink. So she and her husband began to take before-dinner walks. For a half hour to an hour, they strolled around the neighborhood, chatting as they explored the area. She said not only did the walk relax them, but it seemed to keep their appetites at bay so they ate less dinner. A smaller dinner, combined with the exercise, helped them both lose weight. The unexpected bonus, she told me, is that they also sleep better.

5. *Avoid Situations that Make It Hard to Resist Drinking*. We all know that there are certain circumstances that encourage us to drink. Perhaps it's when you get together with a certain friend. Perhaps it's when you play cards with the boys. Maybe you can't resist a beer at a baseball game. You know yourself best. In this first week of not drinking, you're better off avoiding situations that will make it difficult for you to say no. I found when I stopped drinking, that I had to make new friends to replace the ones I had spent evenings drinking with. We no longer had the same interests and I was no longer willing to spend time with them. I found friends who shared my interest in health—many of them were people I met through my new interest in exercise—and it was no longer a struggle to avoid drinking.

Remember, you must avoid drinking completely for only one week and it's not so difficult to miss one card game or one evening out with a friend if you know that could be your downfall. But if you can't avoid the situation, be prepared.

One of my patients was very nervous about attending her sales conference in Florida at the end of her alcohol-free week. Everyone drank liberally at these conferences, and she couldn't imagine attending one without drinking. But, in fact, she handled it beautifully by thinking about every circumstance in which she would be tempted to have a drink. She arrived at the evening cocktail parties forty minutes late so she would only have to spend twenty minutes there. She sipped seltzer, and of course no one knew she wasn't drinking.

As she said, "I don't know why I felt so shy about not drinking. No one even noticed. And I would circulate and was just as happy and talkative as everyone else. When we sat down to dinner I thought I would miss having wine. But I didn't, and everyone was so involved in what they were drinking or eating they never noticed I was just sipping seltzer. I found that I had far more energy and did better at that sales conference than I ever did before. No more of those morning-after agonies when you've really overindulged. And no more worries about doing something regrettable in front of my colleagues. The only thing I missed was the exotic drinks—the piña coladas and margaritas—which are such fun to sip beside the pool when you're relaxing. But all in all I think I was a big success, and I was amazed to notice what a difference not drinking made in my energy level and performance."

The Antialcohol Biochemical Booster

Some people find it more difficult than others to give up drinking entirely, even for one week. Though you should be in good enough physical shape by now—with improved nutrition, no sugar, no caffeine, and with vitamin-mineral supplements—still some of you may need extra help to get through the week. I recommend the supplement glutamine.

A number of years ago Professor William Shive discovered there was a substance that seemed to protect cells to some degree from the ravages of alcohol. It was found in liver extract, cabbage, and high-protein foods like meat, fish, and dairy products. This substance was glutamine, an amino acid. Glutamine seems to help restore the nutritional unbalance that can cause alcoholic cravings in some people. Everybody's body produces glutamine, but some people don't seem to produce enough. If you're one of those people, you may find that a supplement of glutamine will reduce your physical craving for alcohol and will help you get through this week and the rest of the Makeover.

You can get glutamine, called L-glutamine or glutamic acid, in powder form at a health food store. Mix it into fruit juices and drink it. Don't use it in anything hot because heat reduces its effectiveness. I suggest you take 500 milligrams three times a day at meals. Continue to take it for one month. Remember that glutamine is a nutrient and not a drug, so it's perfectly safe.

After Your First Alcohol-Free Week . . .

If you're like most of my patients, you won't have much trouble giving up alcohol for one week. As so many of them have said to me, "After all, I can do most anything for one week." It's the follow-up that's hard.

There are so many temptations to drink, and learning to manage your drinking is, in some ways, more difficult than giving it up completely. Of course, if you decide to stop entirely after this week of the Makeover, that's fine. Only a handful of my patients have made that decision. Most go back to controlled drinking and are pleased to have broken their habit.

After the first alcohol-free week, you can resume drinking, but you have to do so with a different attitude. You can never again drink without thinking. The point is never let yourself fall into a drinking habit again. Drinking can have a role in your life, but you must work to keep it in its place as an occasional pleasure, never a habit. Here are some rules for drinking again after Week Five of the Makeover:

1. *Never Drink Every Night.* This is a hard-and-fast rule. It's drinking every night that builds tolerance and creates a habit difficult to break. I suggest that after your alcohol-free week, you drink only on weekends for the rest of the Makeover. For most people, this means three weeks of weekends-only drinking. Of course, you don't have to drink on weekends, but if a situation arises in which you would enjoy a drink, go ahead and have one. Once you have finished the Makeover, you'll have much less incentive to drink because you'll be very aware of your physical condition, and you'll be less willing to sacrifice even one morning to that sluggish feeling only one or two drinks can cause. If you want to drink during the week after the Makeover, it's perfectly all right as long as you never drink two nights in a row. And as long as you abide by the suggestions that follow.

2. *Never Drink to Relax.* Take a walk, take a bath, do some stretching exercises, have a regular massage. In the next to last week of the Makeover, we'll work on stress and learn some new techniques for relaxing. Use them. Never depend on a drink to mellow you. If you want to have a drink in the evening, relax first, so when

you do have one you are already calm. You'll enjoy it more and you won't be as likely to become dependent on alcohol as a tension releaser.

3. *Notice the Effects of Drink on Your Body*. The new "problem" drinkers usually build up such a tolerance that they don't notice how alcohol affects them. In my case I had been drinking almost every night and, naturally, never noticed how alcohol was affecting me. But when I had spent the week alcohol-free and had a drink on Friday night, Saturday morning came as a slap in the face. It was enormously useful to notice this because it made me realize what I was sacrificing each time I had a drink at night—an energetic, optimistic morning.

Notice the immediate effects of drink on your body. Most of my patients find they've built up far more of a tolerance for alcohol than they had imagined possible. After the alcohol-free week and a few weeks of weekend-only drinking, they discover that one drink has a much stronger effect on them than it used to. Instead of drinking a half-bottle of wine with dinner, they find that just one glass, sipped slowly, gives them a pleasant glow and they have no desire for more. One patient told me that after three weeks of not drinking, she had a glass of wine with dinner and it hit her like Cognac. She felt as if she were a young teenager having her first drink. She was delighted with this reaction, as it helped her limit her consumption and made it much easier for her to avoid letting alcohol become a habit again.

4. *Never Drink to Inebriation*. This is an obvious point. If you drink too much, you'll suffer from a hangover, and a hangover will make it that much more difficult for you to stick to the changes you have already made. You'll feel exhausted, dehydrated, irritable, and headachy. You'll probably crave sweets, and caffeine. You certainly won't feel like exercising. You'll be undoing so much of what you've accomplished.

5. *Count Your Drinks.* This is a simple but effective tactic. When you do drink, pay close attention to how much you're drinking. Don't keep drinking because you feel good and want to maintain that feeling. Your body quickly reaches the point at which it feels best—relaxed, warm, and confident—and after that, everything goes quickly downhill. If you depend only on how you feel and not on the number of drinks, you'll continue to drink until you've had too much.

6. *Drink to Enhance Pleasure.* When you do drink, enjoy it. When drinking becomes routine, it's no fun. Most of the new "problem" drinkers are hardly aware of how much they drink or of how it makes them feel. They drink out of habit. Aside from the health problems they create for themselves, they also rob themselves of enjoyment in the drinking itself. A drink, like a vacation or a rich dessert, should be an occasional part of your life and something you take particular pleasure in. Don't feel guilty about having an occasional drink; make it a pleasurable event.

7. *Don't Drink Under Stress.* Many people believe that a drink will help them forget a problem or deal with it in a relaxed way. This is patently untrue. When you're under stress, alcohol will only exacerbate the difficulty by robbing you of your problem-solving ability. It will also deplete your body of essential nutrients and exhaust its stress-fighting abilities. If you're feeling under pressure, exercise or use the stress-fighting suggestions in Week Seven of the Makeover. They will serve you much better than a drink.

8. *Never Drive If You've Been Drinking.* The information in the beginning of the chapter on the effects of alcohol on your body should be enough to convince you of the hazards of driving after drinking. The growing awareness of this problem has given my patients an excellent excuse not to have a drink on occasions when they feel awkward about refusing it. A few have reported that just explaining that they have to drive is enough to stop overzealous hosts or hostesses from urging them to drink.

Tips from Makeover Veterans

Here are some comments from patients which you might find helpful.

• Barbara Anne H., an executive secretary, told me that she was used to having a drink as soon as she got home after work. She would then sort her mail, prepare dinner, and watch the news. She generally had one more drink with dinner. Barbara Anne found that after she broke her drinking habit, she was able to accomplish much more in the evening. All those little housekeeping chores that seemed too much to attempt after a drink or two were now manageable. She says that this alone was enough incentive to keep her from developing a drinking habit again.

• Bob P., a salesman, entertains customers in the evening. He says his biggest problem was going to bars right after work to have a drink with business associates. He was usually hungry, and his blood sugar and psychological resistance were low. He would munch on the salty snacks that most bars have available to encourage thirst. Of course, these would make him drink more, and he would feel the effect of the alcohol more quickly and strongly on an empty stomach. Now, if he has to entertain after work, he makes sure he has something to eat beforehand. Sometimes, he has just crackers and cheese, or yogurt and fresh fruit. But the food takes the edge off his hunger, and he finds it easier to avoid the bar treats and simply to drink seltzer, if not for the whole evening, at least for most of it. He says that he can usually entertain now on just one drink, even when other people present are having many more than that.

• Mary P., a hard-driving magazine-publishing executive, worked long hours and prided herself on her commitment to the job. Every evening she would have a late dinner followed by three or four drinks. Then she would sink into a chair and watch some late-night television. Mary was really dependent on alcohol to help her relax. After having a few drinks, she knew that she wasn't competent to do any more work; she used alcohol as an excuse for some much-needed relaxation. When Mary thought about how much she drank, she realized the impulse behind her drinking. She felt too guilty just doing nothing, so she took up a hobby—needlepoint. At first, she said it felt odd to do something she had thought of as frivolous, but she realizes now how important it is to help her relax. She has found she looks forward to her needlepoint sessions after dinner, and she still enjoys her late-night television. She rarely drinks now and has far more energy in the morning.

Week Six: Exercise

Exercise—the Linchpin

Adding exercise to your life is one of the most important things you can do to improve your health today and tomorrow. As unrelieved stress seems to be the linchpin that exacerbates all your bad habits and damages your health in far-reaching ways, exercise can be the factor that amplifies all your good habits as it combats the inevitable negative influences on your health. When I tell my patients my convictions about the importance of exercise, many wonder why I make them wait until the sixth week of the Makeover to begin an exercise program. If I could get them to leave my office after a first visit and begin exercising, I surely would do so. But most people aren't psychologically or even physically ready for exercise until this point in the Makeover.

Statistics tell us that about 41 percent of all Americans do not exercise at all. Fifteen to 30 percent exercise sporadically, and only 15 percent exercise regularly. These figures roughly correspond to the levels of exercise among my patients. This means about 85 percent—the people I see in my office and the people who are reading this book—don't exercise at all, or enough. Most of them know they should be exercising. They know, at least in a vague way, what the benefits of exercise are. But they are not doing anything about it. To try and convert these people from a sedentary to an active life right off the bat would be self-defeating. I used to try it, but it never worked. It's just too hard for people to adopt an exercise program simply because they've been told it's good for them.

But now in the sixth week of the Makeover, you are ready for exercise both physically and mentally. You feel more in charge of your body and your health. You're enjoying the benefits of better nutrition. You've eliminated sugar and caffeine from your diet, and your blood sugar is on a more even keel. You've discovered the pleasure of renewed energy and optimism. You're ready to believe that exercise will help you feel better still.

I believe Week Six is one of the most important weeks in the Makeover. Not because of any of the specific results of adopting an exercise program, though they are considerable. But because of the far-reaching effects of exercise on the self-confidence and general sense of well-being experienced by people who exercise. Many of my patients have told me that once they begin to exercise, no matter how simple their adopted program, all the changes they've effected with the Makeover seem that much more important to them. And though most intended to stick with those changes, they find that exercise stiffens their resolve and gives them renewed enthusiasm. Even if you've never managed to stick with any exercise routine in the past, you're going to find that this time things will be different.

This Week's Goal

The goal this week is to become more active. If you already exercise, don't skip this week: You should use it to review your chosen exercise, and see if you're getting all the benefits possible from it. If you don't exercise at all, don't be intimidated by the idea of developing an exercise plan. The point is not to become a world-class athlete or to train for competition. Some of you may find that a program of walking, which you can fit easily into your schedule, will be all the exercise you need. In any case, the important goal this week is to make some progress in developing an exercise routine. By the end of the week you will understand clearly why you should be exercising, and you will have integrated exercise into your life so it has become a habit.

Exercise as Antidote

When I began to exercise, before I experienced my own Makeover, I thought of it as an antidote to all the things I was doing to my body that weren't good for it. If I had been drinking, a good exercise session the next day seemed to "sweat out" the alcohol and I would feel better. If I had eaten too much, the exercise session made me feel as if I were burning off extra calories. A close friend told me that my posture was becoming more and more stooped. He said this during a particularly stressful time in my life, and after his comment I did notice, if I caught a glimpse of myself in the mirror, that I was carrying the weight of the world on my shoulders. So exercise also became an antidote to my deteriorating posture. The program was fairly sporadic. I exercised when I felt I needed to and when I had time.

I used to think of exercise as medicine. It hung over my head like an obligation, and even though I usually enjoyed exercising, I never really thought about it in a positive way. I realize now that my feelings were typical of most people who haven't integrated exercise into their lives. Most people approach exercise as they do taking medicine, and if they maintain that attitude, they have great difficulty sticking with an exercise program.

Exercise as Enhancement

There is another, better way to approach exercise, and it's one I encourage my patients to adopt: exercise as enhancement. Exercise is an enhancement of life, and I believe you need it to feel fully alive. Your body was meant to work, to move, to stretch and sweat. If you allow yourself to take pleasure in using your body, you'll move beyond the exercise-as-antidote attitude and begin to find real joy in your body.

I discovered exercise as enhancement by accident, as many people do. I was never athletic in school. I never thought I would get involved in a serious exercise program. But in the course of developing the Makeover, I began to pay close attention to the effect that exercise was having on me, and I realized that it was making an appreciable difference in my life. Not only was my posture improving, I was feeling stronger and calmer. Best of all, I found I had more energy during the day. This didn't happen all at once: When I first began to exercise, I felt more tired afterward. It was only after a few weeks that I began to notice that exercise was becoming a real enhancement to my life.

I began to research the effects of exercise on the body, and found that my experience was typical. The more I exercised, the more I enjoyed it. Eventually, I competed in a triathlon, a triple-fitness sport involving swimming, bicycling, and running. I was forty-one at the time, and felt more fit than at any other time in my life. I had a greater sense of well-being than I ever had before, and, though at the height of my training I was spending an hour and a half each day exercising, I was accomplishing more on a day-to-day basis than before.

The statistics in a recent Gallup poll reflect my personal experience: People who exercise regularly find that the benefits are greater than they anticipated. In fact, judging from the results of this poll, these benefits are all life-enhancing. Though most of these people began exercising to improve their health (46 percent) or for weight control (24 percent), they also found unexpected benefits:

- They have more energy than they used to (62%)
- Exercise has made them more relaxed (66%)
- Exercise has made them feel more creative at work (43%)
- Exercise has helped them make new friends (46%)

You may begin to exercise for reasons of health and vanity, but if you develop the right program, you'll soon find that exercise touches every area of your life and gives you more pleasure and satisfaction than you had thought possible. The key is to find the right exercise for you, and to stick with it diligently for the rest of the Makeover in order to give it a chance to work. Exercise will no longer be just an antidote, it will be an enhancement.

The Exercise Backlash

Everyone knows that there has been a fitness revolution in this country. You can see it all around you in the celebrity exercise books and the streets filled with joggers. But still there are people who don't exercise and these individuals are looking for excuses. As the commitment to exercise grows, the world becomes divided into two camps: the exercisers and the nonexercisers. The exercisers, according to the current wisdom, have right on their side. The nonexercisers naturally resent them. To add insult to injury, the exercisers seem to be self-absorbed and narcissistic. At least, that's the impression one can get watching them running by or pumping iron at the gym. It's not difficult simply to withdraw from the fray, forget about exercising, and cherish the notion that exercising is a little too trendy for you. But if you do withdraw, you're hurting only yourself. You're reacting to the extreme case, not to the average person who has integrated exercise into his or her life in a simple, reasonable way.

I've noticed this backlash against exercise among my patients. Eva G., a real estate saleswoman, told me that she has become almost proud of ignoring the pressure to exercise. The sixth week of the Makeover took her more than two weeks to accomplish because she was so reluctant to begin exercising. But now Eva realizes she was reacting to the fanatics. As she says, "I'd come to think that exercise meant serious, seven-day-a-week sweating and esoteric equipment, and a wardrobe of exercise fashions, and a mortgage on a gym locker. It was too much for me. But when I realized that I was doing this for me, not for anyone else, and that I could do anything I chose as long as I followed some simple guidelines, the whole project took on a different feeling. I've found three different activities I enjoy—swimming, walking, and bike riding—and I alternate them according to mood and weather. They've been easy to fit into my life and I feel quite silly telling you that I've come to enjoy them so much I haven't missed an exercise session in three months. I'll never be an exercise fanatic, but I love my activities and how they make me feel and look. I've certainly changed my tune about exercise."

The benefits of exercise are real and you can't afford to ignore them. You have to forget about the exercise hype and focus on your own life-style and what exercise can mean to you.

Exercise Incentive

Knowing that exercise is good for you may provide some initial incentive, but it won't keep you going for long. Fortunately, one of the immediate benefits of exercise is also one of the things that will help you stick with it. Exercise enhances your mood. Scientists can't explain how or why it does this, but there's no question it does. Herbert de Vries, professor of physical education at the University of Southern California, tested muscle tension in a group of subjects after half had exercised and half had taken tranquilizers. His study showed that even the minimal exercise that you would get in a fifteen-minute walk is more relaxing than a tranquilizer.

There are various theories on why exercise has this mood-enhancing effect. Some claim exercise increases the levels of certain hormones in the brain, which makes people feel happy. Others have noted that exercise increases the blood supply to the brain, and, based on the fact that senile people who are given oxygen often think more clearly and enjoy improved moods, they think that exercise may similarly improve moods among active people. There's also evidence that beta-endorphins, the body's natural opiates, are produced in high levels when we exercise regularly. Beta-endorphins increase pain tolerance, counter stress, and give an all-around good feeling. Beta-endorphins also help lower blood pressure and suppress appetite, and some researchers have speculated that the production of beta-endorphins is the reason some people become "addicted" to exercise.

Studies have shown that exercise diffuses the Type A personality—the personality that tends to hard-driving competitiveness and to having a chronic sense of urgency, aggressiveness, and even hostility. A Duke University study on forty-six men and women who engaged in a ten-week program of exercise found that scores on tests that measure Type A behavior were reduced significantly.

While an improvement in mood or an ability to relax might not seem like the most important benefit of exercise, I mention it now because it seems to explain why once people begin an exercise program, they are loath to give it up. In fact, one researcher tried to do a study in which thirty people who exercised regularly would discontinue their program for ten weeks, which was the duration of the study. But he couldn't find any regular exercisers who were willing to give up their activity for that long or, for that matter, for any length of time! The point is, once you begin to exercise, no matter how overwhelming the task may seem at the moment, you'll find that your body truly becomes your ally, and the good feelings you derive from exercising will help keep you going.

The Fat Factor: Exercise and Weight

Most of us have grown up with the idea that fat comes from food: The more you eat, the fatter you get. If you cut down on calories, you'll slim down. At the same time, we can't help but recognize that most diets fail. A fast weight loss is often followed by a gain that sometimes surpasses the amount lost. This is the well-known yo-yo effect, and most of us have experienced it.

If weight loss were just a matter of cosmetics, it wouldn't have a role in the Makeover. But obesity is a serious medical problem in this country—62 percent of us are overweight—and it has been directly related to several chronic health problems. Losing weight is secondary to achieving good nutrition (though often the two go hand in hand), but if you are overweight, this is the week to begin trimming down. In Week Three of the Makeover you worked on nutrition, and I made the point that your goal was not to lose weight, but to improve your overall nutrition. Now, this week you'll see how exercise will become the component which, combined with good nutritional habits, will help you to lose weight if you want to.

As diet failure implies, fat does not always come from food. It comes from a "set point," or natural level of fat that your brain and body cells try to achieve naturally. This set-point theory was reported in *The Dieter's Dilemma* by William Bennett, M.D., and Joel Gurin, which stated that your body, much more than your conscious mind, determines how fat you will be. Everyone seems to have an individual set point for a level of fatness that the body strives to maintain. You may starve yourself to below your set point, but you will be stressing your body, and once you go off your diet, you will invariably bounce back to your old overweight state.

If you are overweight, this could be enormously discouraging news because it seems to imply that any efforts to lose pounds permanently are doomed. But that's not the case. Exercise can make the crucial difference. Exercise can help the body achieve a new set point that will allow you to maintain a weight level that looks better on your frame and, of course, is better for your long-term health. Aerobic exercise increases your metabolic rate, increases and helps maintain your lean body weight, and causes enzymatic changes that facilitate fat metabolism. If you are overweight, or would simply like to lose a few pounds, exercise is the answer.

There are a few myths about weight loss and exercise that we should dispel first. Some people believe that exercise isn't worth the effort because it takes too much activity to burn up calories, and if you're not burning calories, you're not losing weight. Putting aside the set-point theory which disproves this myth, other evidence demonstrates that your body burns more calories than usual for hours after you exercise. This is a result of the higher metabolic rate you achieved through exercise. In contrast, dieting will lower the metabolic rate by nearly 20 percent, which means that the dieter, sitting still, is burning fewer calories than the person who just engaged in exercise, even a mild variety. Moreover, the exerciser is burning fat while building or at least preserving muscle, but the dieter is losing a pound of muscle for every three pounds of fat lost.

Finally some people argue that exercise increases their appetite. While it's true that if you play a rousing game of tennis on Saturday morning, and it's your only exercise, you'll probably feel more hungry than usual on Saturday night. But the person who exercises regularly— at least three weekly sessions of aerobic exercise—will find that his appetite is, if not suppressed, at least regulated. Many of my patients have been surprised to find that if they exercise at the end of a working day, their appetite for dinner is diminished. Bob S., a fashion illustrator, told me that he had had to work at sticking with his new nutrition goals until he began to exercise. He would come home in the evening ravenous, and it was a real struggle not to grab some cookies or ice cream in the "sweet boutiques" he passed on his way from the subway. But once he started exercising, he found that he developed a "Zen detachment," as he calls it, from food. It became easy to resist treats and to fix a light, nutritious dinner.

Exercise and Your Heart

Of all the benefits of exercise, perhaps the single most significant, in terms of reducing your risk factors for future disease is that it strengthens your heart and lessens your chance of developing heart disease. Countless studies have shown that the more physically active you are, the less likely you are to suffer a heart attack. Exercise has a beneficial effect on the three greatest heart disease risk factors: blood cholesterol, high blood pressure, and smoking. With regular exercise the blood vessels that feed the heart open wider and the concentration of cholesterol in the blood decreases. As this occurs, you lessen the possibility that clogged vessels will cause a heart attack or a stroke. Moreover, regular exercise encourages the body to form additional blood vessels called "collaterals." These vessels can be called into play if an older vessel becomes clogged, so that the supply of blood is never compromised.

When you exercise, this strengthens the heart muscle so that you have a stronger heart that needs to beat less frequently to provide your tissues with necessary blood. Your heart rate is lower and less likely to raise your blood pressure or send your heart racing when you have to expend energy. In fact, in many cases exercise is all you need to help you lower high blood pressure.

Exercise also decreases the levels of harmful blood fats, like triglycerides and other forms of cholesterol, while it increases the levels of the "good," or HDL (high-density lipoprotein) cholesterols. HDL actually clears cholesterol from the arteries. A Stanford University research team studied a group of sedentary men and discovered that when these men began to run, their HDL levels shot up 16 percent compared with nonactive men.

According to a study at the Tufts University School of Medicine, endurance athletes have thinner blood plasma than sedentary people. Thinner plasma means that the blood moves more easily through the veins, making the job of the heart easier.

Exercise also helps you quit smoking, one of the major risk factors for heart disease. We're going to work on smoking in the last week of the Makeover, but many people find that exercise is just the boost they need to help them quit the habit. They notice how winded smoking makes them, and they begin to feel the good effects of exercise are worth more than the dubious pleasure of lighting up. There is some evidence that exercise decreases the urge to smoke, because the extra oxygen the active person breathes lowers the craving for tobacco.

Fringe Benefits of Exercise

As if improving your mood, helping you lose weight, and reducing your risk of heart disease weren't enough, there are a few other things exercise can do for you.

Osteoporosis is the condition that causes thinning of the bones, particularly in women after menopause, and six to eight million American women suffer from it. But now there is evidence that regular exercise helps maintain the density of the bones and prevents osteoporosis from developing in the first place.

By now you know the dangers of sugar and how a wildly fluctuating blood-sugar level can place stress on your body. Research at the University of California and elsewhere has demonstrated that regular exercise can help you maintain your body's sugar level by making it more responsive to the insulin it secretes. While this is of particular interest to anyone with a family history of diabetes, it also suggests that exercise can be of help to the average person in controlling blood-sugar levels.

Many of my patients are surprised to recognize how exercise helps combat chronic fatigue by increasing their energy levels and capacity for work. It does this by bringing more oxygen to the brain and keeping you more alert during the day. I noticed this was one of the early benefits of my exercise program. At the same time, exercise helps you sleep because it produces beta-endorphins, which help release the day's tension. And, of course, exercise makes you physically tired.

Before You Begin ...

Many people who are planning to start an exercise program wonder if they need medical supervision. I believe that most otherwise healthy people do not. For one thing, I don't believe that all physicians are qualified to determine the best exercise program, even for people who are at risk. My general advice is, if you consider yourself healthy, and your answers to the following quiz don't indicate that you should seek medical advice, then simply proceed. Naturally if you notice any symptoms following exercise or in connection with exercise, you should consult a physician.

Here are some questions, adapted from guidelines of the American Heart Association, that should help you gauge if you have any risk factors that indicate special caution in adopting an exercise program:

1. Have you ever had a heart attack?

2. Have you ever had rapid, irregular heart action or palpitations?

3. Have you ever had pain, pressure, or a tight feeling in your chest during exercise or any physical activity, including sex?

4. Have you ever taken digitalis, nitroglycerin, quinidine, or any other medication for your heart?

5. Have you ever been told by a physician that you have angina pectoris, fibrillation or tachycardia, an abnormal electrocardiogram, a heart murmur, rheumatic heart disease, or any other heart trouble?

• **IF YOU ANSWER YES TO ANY OF THESE QUESTIONS:** There's a high probability that you have a heart problem, either recognized or unrecognized. Before you begin an exercise program, it's essential that you have a complete checkup and probably a stress test. You should exercise only in a medically supervised program—perhaps one run by a cardiologist—with facilities that could handle a heart emergency.

1. Do you have any of the following risk factors for coronary heart disease:
   • Do you have diabetes?
   • Do you have hypertension?
   • Has your physician ever put you on a special diet for your heart or blood pressure, or given you medication to lower your blood cholesterol?
   • Do you have a blood relative who had a heart attack before age sixty?
   • Do you smoke cigarettes?
2. Are you more than twenty pounds overweight?
3. Do you have other health problems that might affect a fitness program, such as chronic illness, asthma, emphysema, or any lung condition, arthritis, rheumatism, or gouty arthritis?
4. Do you get short of breath with activities that don't seem to bother others?
5. Have you ever gotten cramps in your legs if you walk briskly?
6. Do you have any condition limiting the motion of your muscles, joints, or any part of the body, which could be aggravated by exercise?

• **IF YOU ANSWER YES TO ANY OF THESE QUESTIONS:** Before you begin an exercise program, you should have a complete medical checkup and probably a stress test. Depending on the findings of both and the opinion of your doctor, your exercise program could be either supervised or unsupervised. For example, if you have uncontrolled diabetes with constantly fluctuating blood sugar, the diabetes should be under control before you begin any type of exercise program. If you smoke, depending on other health factors and your doctor's opinion, you probably can begin a moderate exercise program without any problem.

Being Realistic

Once my patients are convinced of the need for exercise, they usually want to begin immediately. Most of them want to sign up at a health club or start right in jogging. It's at this point, right at the very beginning, that the novice exerciser is vulnerable to failure. Overenthusiasm can kill your best intentions. Gina M. is a case in point.

Gina came to see me at a friend's suggestion because she was suffering from recurrent headaches and constant exhaustion. She was also overweight by about twenty pounds. It turned out that Gina was a chocolate addict. She also drank an enormous amount of espresso coffee, which she would load with sugar. To compensate for all the chocolate and sugar, which she knew helped keep her fat, she tried to starve herself by never eating breakfast and having just a piece of fruit at lunch. Of course, she often wound up overeating at dinner because she was so hungry.

By the time Gina reached the sixth week of the Makeover, her headaches were gone and she was feeling more energetic. But she was convinced that she would never be able to stick to an exercise program. She had been a member of three different health clubs over a period of years, and had never used one of them more than a half dozen times. She owned a collection of exercise equipment, including leg and arm weights and even a stationary bicycle. Gina had begun each of her efforts with a burst of enthusiasm, but in each instance had tried to do more than she should have. She had joined strenuous exercise classes that ultimately exhausted her, she had tried working with weights that were too heavy for her and even her stationary bicycle, which could have been good exercise, proved overwhelming when she tried to do too many miles for her condition. Gina never knew what shape she was in. She assumed that the more exercise, the better. She was programming herself for failure by taking on more than she could possibly hope to achieve. Instead of having beneficial effects, the exercise was exhausting her physically and discouraging her mentally.

Gina argued that she had already achieved so much on the Makeover that she was satisfied and wanted to skip the exercise week. It took a certain amount of convincing to make her see that she didn't need to undertake a punishing exercise program—that a mild, well-thought-out exercise that she liked and that suited her physical condition would be fun and easy and successful. It turned out that Gina loved swimming, but she didn't think it was "hard" enough to make any difference. Now that she knows how to determine what condition she is in, how to set goals for herself, and how to modify those goals as she makes progress, she realizes that swimming is an excellent exercise, and because she likes it, she has kept to it and is feeling better than she would have thought possible. She has also lost nearly twenty pounds without making any effort to reduce calories.

The Makeover Exercise Goal: Aerobic Fitness

What does it mean to be fit and how can you achieve it? There are three components of physical fitness: endurance, strength, and flexibility. Endurance allows you to produce energy over a long period of time. Strength refers to the amount of force that a muscle can generate.

Flexibility is the range of motion through which a joint can move. Each of these three things is important in any exercise program, but they are not your main goal. Your Makeover goal is simple: You're working toward aerobic fitness. Exercise can have other, very specific goals: working on flexibility with regular stretching exercises, alleviating lower-back pain with calisthenics, or building muscular strength with weight training. You can include these goals in your exercise program, but they should be secondary to aerobic fitness, because aerobic fitness will have the greatest effect on your current feelings of well-being and your ability to handle daily stress, and your prevention of future chronic disease.

What is aerobic fitness? It means the ability of your heart and lungs to support moderately strenuous activity over a period of time. Its goal is to help the heart become a stronger pump that beats less often but pumps more blood. You accomplish this by raising the heart rate during an exercise session and maintaining this elevated heart rate for at least twenty to thirty minutes. There are three principles that neatly summarize this concept of aerobic fitness. They are called the F.I.T. formula and provide a basic outline for how you should exercise.

• FREQUENCY: To really benefit from your exercise, you have to do it often enough that a "training effect" takes place. You must exercise at least three times a week, but I think four times a week is best. You must space your sessions through the week: Don't exercise for three days in a row and then skip four days. If you don't follow a pattern of activity followed by rest days, your body doesn't get a chance to work a muscle and then recover; and if you take too long between exercise sessions, you quickly begin to lose the fitness you've achieved.

• INTENSITY: You must exercise hard enough as well as often enough. How do you know what's hard enough for you? The best way, and the way you're going to depend on, is heart-rate monitoring. You want your heart to beat faster than usual as you exercise—up to a certain point. You want to make extra demands on your heart to increase its power and capacity. It's easy to chart your target heart rate, and I'll show you how in a minute.

• TIME: Finally you have to maintain this higher heart rate for an optimum amount of time. The duration of the exercise is as important as its intensity. If you work in short five-minute bursts of extreme intensity, you won't be getting the cardiovascular benefits of aerobic exercise. I believe the optimum duration of an exercise session is thirty minutes at the beginning. As you progress, you may want to extend the length of the exercise sessions, but it's a mistake to start out with long sessions; they'll tire and discourage you, and you can injure yourself by training too hard at first. Some exercises lend themselves to one-hour periods. That's fine as long as you're working at the proper intensity for your level of training. The point is that you can't reap the benefits of aerobic exercise if the session is shorter than a half hour.

Your Invisible Coach

It's difficult to know how long and how hard to exercise without some specific guidelines. Fortunately, there is an indication of your progress that's totally personal and accurate: your heart rate. Your heart rate is an objective guide and you should become accustomed to taking it regularly to assess your performance. There are three heart rates that count: your resting heart rate, your target heart rate, and your recovery heart rate.

• **YOUR RESTING HEART RATE:** This is your heart rate when you are at rest, and it gives an idea of your general level of physical fitness. If you're in good condition, your heart rate is probably lower than that of someone in poor condition. That's because a fit heart pumps more blood with each contraction and doesn't have to pump as often. The average resting heart rate for women is 78 to 84, and for men, 72 to 78.

• **YOUR TARGET HEART RATE:** This is the rate at which your heart should be beating while you exercise. It indicates your level of cardiovascular fitness. It's the most important heart rate of all. It should guide you in the intensity of your workouts, since you should always be working within your target heart-rate range. If your heart rate while exercising is less than your target heart rate, you're not working hard enough; if it's higher, you're working too hard.

Here's how to figure out your target heart rate:

220 minus your age (____) = (your maximum heart rate)

Your maximum heart rate (____) multiplied first by .7 = your minimum target heart rate (____)

Your maximum heart rate multiplied by .85 = your maximum (____) target heart rate.

For example, if you are thirty-six years old, your maximum heart rate is 220 minus 36, or 184. The number 184 multiplied by .7 and .85 equals 128 and 156. Therefore, 128 to 156 is the range of your target heart rate. Depending on your level of fitness (which you'll figure out using the Modified Step Test in the next section), you should be working at either the high or the low end of your target heart rate.

• **YOUR RECOVERY HEART RATE:** This is the heart rate taken five minutes after you've stopped exercising. It indicates how quickly you recover. As you continue to exercise, your heart will become stronger and your recovery heart rate will drop. If the count is greater than 120 beats per minute, you've been working too hard and you should cut down on the intensity of your workout.

How to Take Your Heart Rate

You need a watch or clock with a second hand. Find your pulse either on the thumb side of your wrist or the side of your neck, just next to your windpipe. Don't use your thumb for locating your pulse because it has its own strong pulse, which can throw off the count. As you watch the second hand, count your pulse for exactly six seconds. Multiply that number by ten to get your heart rate per minute.

Taking Stock: You and Your Heart

If you want to be realistic about your exercise program, you have to know what kind of shape you're in right now, so you can tell if you should be working at the high or low end of your target heart rate. This information will help you set goals for the future. I suggest that you take the following Modified Step Test, which will help you gauge your current fitness level. You'll need a stopwatch to time yourself and a step stool or a bench that is eight inches high. Don't take this step test if your responses to the quiz on page 236 indicate that you may have a heart problem.

The Modified Step Test

1. Ask someone with a stopwatch or one with a sweep second hand to time you.
2. At the signal to begin, step up (start with either foot) on a stair, stepstool, or bench that is 8 inches from ground level, and step down again. Continue stepping up and down, alternating feet, for 3 consecu-

tive minutes at a rate of 24 steps per minute—about 2 steps every 5 seconds.

3. Stop at exactly 3 minutes and immediately sit down in a chair. The active part of the test is now completed.

4. At exactly 1 minute after you completed the test, count your pulse for 15 seconds and multiply by 4 to obtain your 1-minute pulse-recovery score.

5. Refer to the following table to determine the rating for your score. If you are unable to do the exercise for the full 3 minutes, consider your aerobic fitness poor.

Ratings for the Modified Step Test

The scores below are for heartbeats per minute, measured one minute after completion of the Modified Step Test. Ratings for scores are based on age and sex.

Age	Very High	High	Moderate	Low	Very Low
Female					
10–19	below 82	82–90	92–96	98–102	above 102
20–29	below 82	82–86	88–92	94–98	above 98
30–39	below 82	82–88	90–94	96–98	above 98
40–49	below 82	82–86	88–96	98–102	above 102
50–59	below 86	86–92	94–98	100–104	above 104
60–69	below 86	86–92	94–98	100–104	above 104
Male					
10–19	below 72	72–76	78–82	84–88	above 88
20–29	below 72	72–78	80–84	86–92	above 92
30–39	below 76	76–80	82–86	88–92	above 92
40–49	below 78	78–82	84–88	90–94	above 94
50–59	below 80	80–84	86–90	92–96	above 96
60–69	below 80	80–84	86–90	92–96	above 96

Assessing Your Modified Step Test Score

If you are sedentary, your score will probably be around 100 or above, no matter what your age. Conversely, if you are exceptionally fit, your score will be below that of someone your age who is less fit. If your score on the Modified Step Test is well below 100—falling under the high or very high ratings—you have a high cardiorespiratory recovery rate and are aerobically very fit. Chances are you exercise regularly. Keep it up. A moderate or low rating indicates there is room for improvement in your aerobic fitness. If your score falls within the very low rating, then a regular exercise program could make a big difference in your day-to-day energy level as well as in your long-term health.

The results of the Modified Step Test will give you an idea of how quickly your heart recovers from exercise. It tells you how strong your heart is, and gives you a baseline from which to proceed when judging the effectiveness of an exercise program. The sooner your heart rate returns to its resting rate, the better your condition. Your pulse rate should come down to around 120 within five minutes after you stop exercising, and it should be down to 100, or lower, within ten minutes. If you're in good shape, your rate will drop below 100 within five minutes. Make sure to keep a note of your rating, so that you can repeat the test in a few weeks to determine how much progress you're making.

Choosing Your Exercise

This is the one part of the Makeover where you're on your own. I can't tell you which exercise is best for you. One of the most important aspects of the exercise you choose, aside from being one that fulfills the F.I.T. requirements, is that you enjoy it. I've learned that the only patients who have trouble sticking to their exercise programs are those who choose something they don't really enjoy—they still view exercise as medicine. It's essential that you avoid this.

Remember that there's no hard-and-fast rule about staying with a single exercise program. Many people think that they have to choose one type of exercise and do it three or four times a week. For some people, this works best because it eliminates decision making, which could make it easy to skip an exercise session; but others find that they enjoy having two or three different exercises which they do on alternate days. You may want to let the weather determine what exercise you engage in. One of my patients rides a stationary bicycle in bad weather and jogs on nice days. The key to choosing the right program is knowing yourself and knowing what you'll be able to stick with.

Here are the four most popular aerobic exercises. The majority of my patients choose one of these as the basis for their programs:

• RUNNING AND JOGGING: These are the most popular aerobic exercises because you can do them anywhere, they don't require expensive equipment, and they are among the most efficient in terms of calories burned for time spent exercising. (By the way, if it takes you more than eight minutes to run a mile, you're a jogger; less than that, you're a runner.) It has been documented that jogging and running result in the fastest weight loss of all aerobic exercises, though this shouldn't be the sole reason for taking them up. Many of my patients enjoy jogging and have found it easy to incorporate it into their daily routine. There are some cautions about jogging mainly having to do with injury. Running is hard on your legs and feet, and there's no doubt that it increases the incidence of joint trauma. The force on your feet is about three times your body weight. If you have orthopedic or joint problems, consult your doctor before you begin to run. And everyone who begins a running program should be sure to wear running shoes that fit properly. If you're interested in running as an exercise, I suggest that you get one of the many books available on the subject.

• **WALKING:** I think walking is the most underrated exercise. Many of my patients who never thought they would have the time to do an enjoyable exercise have begun a program of walking that has proven successful. Most people don't realize that for every mile you walk you burn the same number of calories as for miles run. One mile equals about 100 calories whether you walk or run. It just takes you longer to walk. The only caution if you choose walking as an aerobic exercise is that you must be sure that your heart rate is within your target range. You must walk briskly enough to raise your pulse for the required half hour. Some people find that they need to carry some weight in order to do this. You can wear a backpack with a few books in it or simply carry hand weights. Many of my patients walk to work as their aerobic exercise, and find that carrying a briefcase gives enough extra weight to raise their pulse to the right level. If you begin walking as an aerobic exercise, be sure you wear comfortable, well-fitting shoes.

• **CYCLING:** This is an excellent aerobic exercise—I got interested in it when I trained for the triathlon. I began cycling on weekends in the country. I found it exhilarating and soon began a serious training program. Cycling four miles is equivalent to running one mile. Under the best conditions, the injury rate is lower than that for running. But some of you will never find the best outdoor conditions, because if you bike on city streets, you're competing with traffic, which can be very dangerous, and it may be difficult to find a nonstop route that will allow you to maintain your target heart rate. Even if you cycle in the country or on quiet streets, be sure to wear a helmet and protective kneepads. Some of my patients cycle outdoors on weekends and in good weather, and use a stationary bike in bad weather. Stationary bikes provide the same cardiovascular benefits as outdoor bikes, and you can adjust the resistance on the bike to make it easier to maintain your target heart rate. But I don't recommend basing your program entirely on using a stationary bike, as most people who try to do this become bored very quickly. I recommend it as an alternative to outdoor biking.

• **SWIMMING:** Swimming is a good aerobic exercise, and it will help tone and strengthen the muscles in your arms and legs. A big advantage to swimming is that it doesn't put the strain on your joints, legs, and feet that jogging or even cycling can. It's a rhythmic activity that uses the most muscle groups of all aerobic exercises. It's very gentle. The drawback to swimming is that you must really work at it: Swimming for cardiovascular fitness is not at all like taking a dip in a pool while on vacation. You have to be sure you're working to your target heart rate for at least a half hour. Swimming also burns fewer calories per minute than running.

Here are a few other suggestions for aerobic exercises that my patients have adopted successfully as at least part of an overall program:

• **CROSS-COUNTRY SKIING:** This is an excellent aerobic exercise because not only do you use your entire body (including the upper body, which running does not), but it is also great fun. It burns a lot of calories—485 per hour—and is one of the best cardiovascular exercises known. In fact, some of the highest oxygen consumption levels recorded have been among cross-country skiers. Of course, it's a seasonal exercise for most people, and it does require a bit of training.

• **AEROBIC DANCING:** A few of my patients have found that aerobic dancing classes have been the perfect solution to their aerobic exercise needs. Unlike running or walking, aerobic dancing uses all the muscles of your body. My patients claim, however, that its biggest appeal is that it's fun and it's social. They are loath to miss a class because they really enjoy the activity.

• **CALISTHENICS:** Doing calisthenics at home on your own can sometimes be difficult: It's just too easy to skip a session. But many people find that the best way to integrate exercise into their lives is to join a gym and take calisthenics. If you choose calisthenics, keep track of your target heart rate as you exercise and let it be a guide to the intensity of your workouts.

Sticking with It

The hardest part of an exercise program is facing the second or third week. Usually you can get through the first week on sheer enthusiasm. But as the days go by, something always comes up as an appealing alternative to the exercise session. And then if you skip once, you'll be tempted to skip again; and before you know it, a whole week has gone by and you haven't exercised once. If you can manage to stick with the program for the first three weeks, you'll probably find, like most of my patients, that you'll look forward to it because you recognize how good it makes you feel. But in the beginning, it takes simple willpower to keep going. Here are some tips from Makeover veterans, and from my own experience, that should help keep you on track:

• **CHOOSE SOMETHING YOU ENJOY:** This is perhaps the single most important step you can take to ensure a successful exercise program. You can be certain you won't continue with any workout that you don't enjoy. Don't think that this time it will be different; it won't. If you don't look forward to doing the exercise, it's just too easy to find an excuse to avoid it. The biggest danger after you begin is boredom; and the more you can do to avoid being bored, the better your chances of success. One of my patients, Suzanne K., who is a children's-book illustrator, was discouraged about finding an exercise she liked. She hated gyms and jogging and most other popular physical activities. But when I asked her what her fantasy exercise would be, she answered without hesitation: ballet. It had never occurred to her to take classes because she was too old and because she had never taken any ballet lessons before. It wasn't difficult to find a class that was right for her and she's delighted she did. She told me that the class means a lot to her, not only because of the exercise, which makes her feel wonderful, but also because it's something she had always dreamed about doing but had never dared try.

• **SET A REGULAR EXERCISE SCHEDULE:** The main reason people give for not exercising is lack of time. But the busiest people can find the time to exercise during the week if they set it as a priority. It's been my experience that if you plan to exercise "when you have time," you never will. We all lead busy lives, and sometimes the pressure to do other things can seem overwhelming. You need to have a regular exercise schedule to keep you on track. I schedule my exercise sessions for after work, and I view them as important appointments in my day; I would no sooner skip a session than skip an appointment with a patient. Exercising after work helps me relieve the tension of the day, and it also reduces my appetite so that I eat a lighter meal in the evening. Some people find that early-morning exercising gives them a boost of energy that lasts throughout the day. You have to decide what time is physically and psychologically the best for you. One warning: Some people find that if they exercise late in the evening they are too revved up to sleep. If this happens to you, reschedule your exercise session for earlier in the day.

• **MAKE EXERCISE FUN:** Do anything possible to add pleasure to the sessions. Exercise with music, or to a favorite television show. Get a tiny radio-cassette player that you can listen to while you run or ski or dance. One of my patients discovered that the best way to stick with his exercise program is to work out while watching the evening news. He watched the news anyway, so it was easy to exercise at the same time. The news keeps him interested, and from having to decide every evening when to exercise and whether or not he should.

• **MAKE EXERCISE CONVENIENT:** If you plan to play tennis, but the courts are miles from your house, or if you want to swim, but the pool is only open a few hours each week, you're creating a problem for yourself. The more inconvenient it is to get to your exercise class, the less likely you will do so. One of my patients told me that she had joined a gym and planned on going three times a week. As she worked at home and the classes were at convenient times, she thought this would be an effective program. But the gym was far enough away that it took her over a half hour to get there. The class itself was an hour, and when she added changing and shower time, each exercise session took over three hours. After a few weeks, she realized that she couldn't devote so much time to exercising during the day and expect to keep up with her work. You have to be realistic. A dance class around the corner may be a better solution than an exercise class at a gym on the other side of town.

• **DON'T GET BORED:** You have to guard against boredom no matter what exercise you choose. If you run or walk, change your route regularly. If you do calisthenics, change the number of repetitions or try some different exercises. Buy a new tape to listen to while you dance. If you get bored with your exercise class, change to a new one.

• **EXERCISE WITH A FRIEND:** This can be an excellent way to keep up the momentum. But you must be sure your friend is as committed to exercise as you are. If he or she skips too many sessions, your determination will waver. On the other hand, a friend who is enthusiastic can be a boon. It makes exercise fun and keeps your interest level high. Someone who expects you to exercise a few times a week can also put just the amount of pressure on you that you need to stick with your program.

• **TRICK YOURSELF INTO GETTING STARTED:** One of my patients told me that she sometimes found it almost impossible to get out to run in the morning. Finally she devised a system: On days when she really didn't want to get moving, she told herself that she would run only one quarter of her usual distance and use the extra time to read the paper before work. She discovered that once she got started, she always ran the full distance because she enjoyed it so much. But if she thought about that full distance as she was trying to get out of bed, she knew she would never make it. Do anything you can to get yourself started. Tell yourself you'll only do a portion of your exercise, or promise yourself a treat when you finish.

• **BUY BOOKS FOR INSPIRATION:** It's almost inevitable that you'll get stale at some point. I suggest you buy a book about your particular exercise and read it for inspiration. If there's a magazine devoted to your exercise, subscribe to it. This can be just the jolt you need to psych yourself to further efforts.

Week Seven: Stress Control

This is the week that's going to tie together the Makeover for you and help complete your leap into vital good health. If you don't smoke, it's the last week of what I hope is your new and better life-style. It's a critical week because learning to control stress is not only going to help fulfill the promise of the Makeover—a healthier and more vigorous life right now as well as in the future—it's going to enable you to stick with the changes you've made for months and years to come.

Stress could be your most serious health problem because it affects every aspect of how your body works. If you have a tendency to headaches, stress will increase their occurrences. If you have a tendency to cardiovascular disease, stress will increase your risk. Even if you're in excellent health—and by now you're feeling better than you have for years—uncontrolled stress will keep you from reaching your full potential physically and mentally. Of course, the converse is true: When you get stress under control, this amplifies the good achieved by each change you've made during the Makeover.

In addition to the important physical benefits of stress

control, there's a psychological bonus that you'll enjoy as soon as you begin this week. I call it the "confidence factor." As soon as you learn to control everyday stress, you'll notice a welcome boost in your self-confidence. Many of my patients have remarked on this exciting benefit of stress control. As you learn how to get on top of the nagging problems that used to wear you out, make you sick, and keep you from performing at your best, you'll also learn how to focus your energy in a positive way to turn stress to your advantage. Therefore, this week represents an effort to control your *life* as well as the stress in it. By the end of the week you'll be a calmer, more effective person—someone who, as one of my patients said, feels "ready and eager for anything that comes my way."

Barb H., a computer saleswoman, had an interesting comment on the positive aspects of stress control. Barb came to see me because she suffered from eczema, which had disappeared for years only to return when she began a demanding job at a new midtown computer store. "I knew there was stress in my life. I believed I could probably do something about it. But I never believed it would make much of a difference. Only when you practically forced me to deal with stress in the Makeover did I come to understand what you'd been saying all along. While I wasn't surprised that the stress was making the eczema flare up, I would never have thought that I could do something as simple as a few exercises to make it disappear.

"Yes, now I feel more relaxed in stressful situations. Yes, my eczema is gone. And yes, I've found the techniques helpful in keeping me away from the junk-food binges that I used to go on. But what I never expected is that I'd feel more in control of my life than ever before. I don't get a knot of anxiety when I have to deal with a demanding client. I don't shy away from making difficult phone calls. I wouldn't say I'm more assertive, but I'm able to peel away the layers of emotion that used to be part of any kind of confrontation. It's not only made these situations easier for me, it's made me infinitely more effective at work. People notice the new me. And in the crazy, competitive world of computers a calm, sound voice is appreciated. I would never have guessed that this week of the Makeover would make the biggest difference of all."

This Week's Goal

In the beginning of the Makeover, we talked in detail about the effects of stress on the body and how it interferes with many aspects of good health. But now we're going to focus on the practical: How you can save yourself from the damage of stress, how you can sometimes avoid it, and how you can often turn it to your advantage. You're going to learn two simple exercises that will help combat the physical damage it causes. The exercises are easy, and the time they demand minimal, but you'll find that they make an amazing difference in how you feel. In addition to the exercises, you'll learn some special methods for coping with difficult people and situations. These methods are in the form of stress tips at the end of the chapter. These tips will free you from the mental baggage that makes you a victim of stress.

Because stress is the "invisible illness," this week we're going to learn how to make it visible. You'll learn to recognize its visible symptoms. When you realize the many ways stress can make itself evident, you'll be even more convinced of the important role it plays in your health. And because everyone's reaction to stress is highly individual, you're going to learn to become aware of your own reactions and be sensitive to your personal symptoms.

There are three simple facts you need to know about

stress, and I hope to convince you of them this week:

• *Uncontrolled stress is killing you*. It is really worse than you think. Stress exacerbates every health problem and increases every health risk you live with.

• *You can control stress*. No matter how frantic and demanding your life and work, you don't have to be a victim of stress. You can cope successfully with it, and sometimes even turn it to your advantage by achieving a new perspective on your everyday problems and conflicts.

• *Controlling stress will change your life as well as your health*. Remember that uncontrolled stress inhibits your potential for happiness as well as for good health. Controlling stress doesn't just make you feel calmer, it makes you feel more in control of every aspect of your life.

You have a head start in controlling stress. Many of the changes you've made during the Makeover have given you a physiological advantage. You've improved your nutrition; you've eliminated caffeine, sugar, and alcohol—all of which are stress triggers; you've begun exercising; and you've initiated a program of vitamin and mineral supplements, including those geared specifically to fighting stress.

All these efforts have given your body ammunition to fight the effects of stress. But unless you come to grips with stress directly, you'll find that over time it will weaken your resolve. Despite your newfound vigor, your life is still filled with pressures. Eventually, you'll have an extraordinarily stressful day and you'll yearn for a drink or a cigarette or a bag of Oreos. Mastering stress after conquering your other bad habits will give you the strength to continue in your new, healthy life-style. Effective stress management improves your feelings of self-control and permeates every aspect of life. It will help you to stick to the changes you've made in the course of the Makeover and enjoy far-reaching health benefits for years to come.

Do You Recognize the Stress in Your Life?

When I ask my patients if they're under stress, many of them answer, "Sure, but it's not bothering me." In fact, these people, like so many, are ignorant of the ways in which stress takes it toll. Here are some questions that will help you recognize the symptoms of stress:

1. Have you been having trouble falling asleep?
2. Have you been waking at night and finding it difficult to get back to sleep?
3. Have you been more short-tempered lately?
4. Have you been feeling anxious for no particular reason?
5. Do you find it difficult to relax?
6. Have you been feeling irritable and easily upset?
7. Have you been working harder than usual?
8. Do you feel that you have more and more to do and less and less time in which to do it?
9. Do you find you're more tired than usual, even after sleep?
10. Has there been a change for the worse in your health?
11. Have you been having more arguments with your spouse lately?
12. Have you been feeling particularly moody?
13. Have you been drinking more coffee, tea, or soft drinks in an effort to keep your energy level up?
14. Have you been smoking more than usual?
15. Have you been craving more sweets than usual?
16. Have you been drinking more alcohol than usual?

If you answered yes to three or more questions, you may be a victim of stress. The symptoms pinpointed in these questions signal the fact that stress has caused a change in your biochemistry. Your ability to cope with stress has been compromised and you could be more likely to develop more serious medical problems.

Stress Risks

In the beginning of the Medical Makeover, I talked about stress being the linchpin that links habit and disease. That earlier chapter on stress was devoted to its physiology: precisely what it is and how your body reacts biochemically. I discussed the link between stress and blood sugar, and how stress chains you to your bad habits, weakens your willpower and causes many diseases in both the short and long terms. That chapter should have convinced you of the dramatic and pervasive effect stress has on your body.

Here are some concrete examples of how stress can work on the mind to affect the body. Animal research has shown in a dramatic way what this can do. For example, mice flown from Boston to Seattle took three days to recover from dangerous levels of adrenaline, cortisol, and other body chemicals. The stress of the flight—the unfamiliar movement, noise, and temperature changes—had aroused the fight-or-flight response in the mice, yet they were captives of their situation. They had no way to discharge these chemicals. Another, more poignant example of the danger of stress was an experiment involving Hamadryas baboons, which form strong lifetime attachments to their mates. Researchers split up baboon couples, putting the males in separate cages but within view of their mates. New males were placed in the females' cages. Within six months the displaced male baboons suffered all the symptoms of heart disease: Some developed high blood pressure, some had heart attacks, and some died of sudden cardiac arrest.

These animal studies and countless others with humans demonstrate that the brain is capable of turning on the body when we are under unrelieved stress. To condense and simplify the process described earlier in this book: Stress causes measurable changes in bodily functions. Your body prepares for fight or flight by releasing the stress hormones epinephrine and norepinephrine, which speed the heart rate and constrict blood vessels. On a physical level, your blood pressure and heart rate increase; emotionally you feel tense and irritable.

The increased blood pressure caused by constant stress is its most dangerous side effect. High blood pressure is one of the three major causes of atherosclerosis. If you don't control the stress in your life, you dramatically increase your chances of having a heart attack or a stroke. In fact, uncontrolled stress is a prime risk factor in heart disease. It is as important, if not more so, than smoking, high blood pressure, and raised blood-cholesterol levels in determining your chances of heart disease. It has been estimated that deaths traced to high blood pressure account for more than half of the deaths in this country every year. Moreover, varying degrees of hypertension, or high blood pressure, are present in 15 percent to 33 percent of the adult population. Tragically hypertension can be a silent killer, since you can suffer for years with no symptoms.

As discussed in the earlier chapter, stress has also been linked to cancer, ulcers, asthma, a wide range of emotional difficulties, and a lowered resistance to infectious diseases because of damage to the immune system. For example, studies have shown that stress in the home can increase a child's risk of streptococcal throat infections. One very revealing recent study assessed pregnant women, married, of similar age, race, and social status, all of whose babies were delivered in the same hospital. The finding: Those women undergoing a great deal of social stress and lacking strong social supports—measured by closeness of ties with husband, family, and community— had almost three times the frequency of complications of pregnancy or delivery. Some very common results of stress that my patients complain of include headaches, insomnia, irritability, impotence, and depression.

Finally stress hinders long-term health by making you more prone to the very bad habits that the Makeover works to change. Some people reach for a cigarette when they're nervous; some go on eating binges. One woman patient would eat an entire bag of cookies after a stressful day at work. As I pointed out earlier, these bad habits reinforce one another: A sweet snack will eventually cause a drop in your blood sugar that will make you yearn for a cup of coffee as a pick-me-up; a drink may make you crave a cigarette. All these are ineffective and ultimately dangerous ways of dealing with stress. When you learn how to cope with stress effectively, it will be easier to resist cigarettes, alcohol, caffeine, and sweets because your body won't suffer the wild fluctuations of blood sugar that make you yearn for bogus energy producers.

The "Escape Myth"

You can't eliminate the stress in your life. It is a component of normal living, and indeed a certain amount of stress is valuable to enable you to adapt to changing circumstances. But the kind of stress most of us endure in our daily lives is ultimately, literally, killing. Many of my patients, and, in fact, many of the people I know, believe that if only they could escape to another, simpler life, they would be stress-free, much healthier and happier. They imagine themselves living in a small town or on a farm, safe from the demands of high-pressure urban life. I want you to stop and decide if you are a believer in this "escape myth." If you are, recognize and discard the belief now because it will keep you from taking this week seriously, and it will interfere with the successful control of stress.

The escape myth, in my opinion, is almost as damaging as the stress itself. Why? Because when we believe that someday we'll flee from our problems to another world, we're tacitly accepting the idea that it's impossible to do anything about those problems today. We come to accept the notion that there's nothing we can really do about the stress in our lives, so we'll just grin and bear it until we can finally escape it entirely.

The escape myth also ignores a fact of human personality. As I said in the beginning of this chapter, it's how you personally react to stress that's important. Even the most ardent believers in the escape myth must admit there's no escaping their personalities. Stress-prone people are going to suffer as much when the well runs dry or the chickens don't lay as they did back in the city from the crime rate or from their bosses' unreasonable expectations.

Maureen D., a nurse in a Manhattan hospital, was a patient. I remember her well because, as a health professional, she was very aware of the toll stress was taking on her. After all, she saw patients every day who were suffering from the long-term effects of unrelieved stress, and it scared her. Maureen decided that she had a bad case of burnout. She was always exhausted and was beginning to think about quitting her job because she felt she could no longer cope with the demands of her patients and her superiors. She said she resented every time she heard the buzzer ring at the nurses' station even though she felt genuine compassion for her patients.

Maureen was a typical believer in the escape myth. She was convinced job stress had forced her into a corner. Because she knew that this pressure was affecting her health, she thought it was necessary to quit. As sophisticated as she was about health-related matters, it never occurred to her to try to alleviate the stress, even though she knew there were effective methods for stress control.

Maureen began to work on stress-control exercises right at the beginning of her Makeover because it was obvious that stress was a serious problem jeopardizing her career. After a month, she told me that she felt like a different person. The change in her feelings about her work was particularly gratifying. Even though the job hadn't changed, and even though we had never worked on reducing the stress itself, the relaxation exercises on page 271 had completely transformed the way she dealt with the stress and had given her a tranquillity that pervaded every aspect of her life.

The danger of the escape myth is that it makes you believe that you must avoid stress in order to feel well. Of course, you can't avoid stressful situations. You need to learn instead how to control your reactions to them so that you can short-circuit the physiological damage to your health.

Stress Buildup

If you think of yourself as immune to the damaging effects of stress, you're probably suffering more than usual. In my experience, the person who prides himself or herself on working well under pressure, or staying cool in a crunch, is the one most liable to sustain long-term damage from stress. These people steel themselves to take on more and more stress, and greater and greater damage results.

Stress buildup is a common syndrome among career-oriented people. They believe they can handle much more pressure today than they could a few years ago. But many of these people simply don't recognize their own symptoms of stress. Chronic headaches, fatigue, increased smoking, back pain, gassiness, cold feet, and premenstrual tension are just a small sampling of these symptoms. Many people never connect these ailments with stress.

But what is most troublesome is that stress buildup ultimately threatens your long-term health. If you try to adapt physically and mentally to ever-increasing amounts of stress without compensating for them, you may not suffer the effects today or tomorrow, but surely at some point in the future you will pay the price with chronic disease. Remember that high blood pressure, for example, is particularly dangerous because it is symptomless. Ulcers and heart disease are just two problems you could be developing unknowingly while you pride youself on your ability to "handle stress." And finally, of course, stress buildup takes its toll on your feelings of contentment and your ability to take pleasure in everyday activities.

Mary Jane H., a reporter with a major city newspaper, is an excellent example of someone who had stress buildup. She came to see me because of chronic fatigue. Mary Jane had been promoted twice in the past year to jobs with ever-increasing responsibilities. After the first promotion, she began to notice that she felt exhausted every afternoon. She was basically happy with her work, but she admitted that she was anxious about doing well and lately she had been wondering if she had chosen the right career. Was the pressure really worth it? After her second promotion, her fatigue increased to the point where it was all she could do to stay awake in the late afternoon. By then she had ten people reporting to her, and felt the pressure not only to reach her job goals, but also to manage her staff effectively. Though she never told anyone at work, she began to think about leaving her job and going to law school.

Over a period of a year, Mary Jane had gradually become accustomed to ever-increasing amounts of stress so that it felt normal to her. But her body as well as her spirits was rebelling. Her constant exhaustion was the only physical symptom. A generalized depression about her work troubled her even more. Once Mary Jane recognized that her stress load had increased dramatically in just one year and that she had done nothing to control it, she understood that her fatigue was not so mysterious and began to see that she had been letting stress get the better of her. As soon as she realized that she could control the stress and even turn it to her advantage, she began to see her job in a new light. She no longer felt "condemned" to her work, but rather saw herself in control of both it and her life.

Moving into the Week

It's time to learn how to cope with stress in your life. I have developed a four-point plan that's simple and effective. First, you'll discover how you yourself react to stress. You'll learn an easy relaxation exercise, done twice daily, that will help defuse stress. You'll learn what triggers the stress in your life. And you'll learn a quick-fix stress reliever.

Your Personal Reaction to Stress

The single most important thing you should know is how to measure your own stress tolerance by becoming sensitive to stress symptoms. While no one is immune, some people react more strongly to stressful situations than others and have more powerful biochemical changes that ultimately do more harm to their bodies.

There have been many efforts to quantify the effects of stress on our bodies. Dr. Meyer Friedman and Dr. Ray Rosenman's trailblazing book, *Type A Behavior and Your Heart*, was one such effort. And you've probably seen one version of a "stress rating list" that categorizes stress by number, allotting, say, 100 points to the death of a spouse and 60 points to divorce. I think that these studies are useful because they help point out the varieties of stressors in our lives and the ways in which different people react to them. But I don't think they're very practical. You have only to pause and reflect for a moment to see that divorce may be a wrenching nightmare for one person but a long-awaited liberation for another. The "mortgage over $10,000" stressor which is often cited on such lists may be a trifle for someone with a six-figure income and an inspiration for ulcers for a person who's unemployed.

Far more important than quantifying stress is finding its role in your life. I've adapted the list of Type A behavior patterns described by Drs. Friedman and Rosenman, not to help you decide if you're a Type A, but rather to help you become more sensitive to behavior patterns that indicate a high susceptibility to stress. Read through the list below and see if any of these behaviors apply to you. If they do, you must look especially carefully for the stress symptoms, which I'll discuss shortly, even if you think that you cope well with stress or don't have much of it in your life.

1. Scheduling more and more activities into less and less time.

2. Failing to notice or be interested in the environment or things of beauty.

3. Hurrying the speech of others.

4. Becoming unduly irritated when forced to wait in line or when driving behind a car you think is moving too slowly.

5. Gesticulating when you talk.

6. Frequent knee jiggling or rapid tapping of your fingers.

7. Explosive speech patterns or frequent use of obscenities.

8. Making a fetish of always being on time.

9. Having difficulty sitting and doing nothing.

10. Playing nearly every game to win, even when playing with children.

11. Measuring your own and others' success in terms of numbers (e.g., number of business deals concluded, articles written, etc.).

12. Lip clicking, head nodding, fist clenching, table pounding, and sucking in air when speaking.

13. Becoming impatient when watching others do things you can do better or faster.

14. Rapid eye blinking or tic-like eyebrow lifting.

While it's important to recognize the behaviors associated with stress, I think it's considerably more important to recognize the symptoms of stress. These symptoms are clear signals that something is wrong, and, although you may not find them dramatic, their implications are ominous for your health.

Here is a rundown of common stress signals, divided into physical, emotional, and behavioral categories. Please read this list carefully. Learning to recognize these symptoms is the key to success for this week.

Physical Symptoms

oiliness of skin
cold hands
sweaty hands
cold feet
sweaty feet
burping
gassiness
need to urinate
diarrhea
tight or tense muscles
acid stomach

palpitations
face flushes
trembling hands
shallow, rapid breathing
shortness of breath
pain in neck or lower back
dryness of throat and mouth
headaches
premenstrual tension
missed periods
exhaustion
elevated blood pressure

Emotional Symptoms

boredom, dullness, general lack of interest
depression
listlessness
constant fatigue
sense of unreality, weakness, fear
inability to concentrate
urge to cry or run or hide
irritability
feelings of hyperexcitation or mania
nightmares
feelings of impending doom
general feelings of resentment
apathy
general feelings of powerlessness
loneliness

Behavioral Symptoms

nail biting
teeth grinding
stuttering or speech difficulties
increased smoking
increased use of drugs or alcohol

Behavioral Symptoms (continued)

decreased or increased eating
insomnia
loss of enthusiasm and/or sense of humor
constant hair pulling or twisting
accident-proneness
high-pitched or unprovoked laughter
trembling or nervous tics
clutching something tightly
foot jiggling
efforts to withdraw and/or isolate yourself

Do you suffer from any of these symptoms? Most of my patients find that they exhibit three to a dozen of them at various times. Check off the ones that apply to you and during this week reread the list a few times. Throughout the week, notice any symptoms as they occur. When you become familiar with the effects that stress is having on your body, you're ready to practice the coping exercises and also to turn stress to your advantage whenever possible.

Relaxation and Stress

Most people's ideas about what constitutes real relaxation do them more harm than good. When I ask my patients what they do to combat stress, I usually get the same answers: "I play softball on weekends to relax," "I go sailing," "I collapse in front of the TV every evening." Most of them suffer from the mistaken notion that this kind of relaxation combats stress. But the relaxation they're describing is just another activity—more agreeable and pleasurable than work, perhaps, but another activity nonetheless. Unfortunately, people who think that these diversions are "relaxing" are getting no stress relief at all, because they believe they have their stress problems under control.

The worst remedies to combat stress are the most popular. They include alcohol, drugs, and cigarettes. While it's true that these solutions will provide temporary "relaxation," in the long run they do far more harm than good by compounding the bad effects of stress. Of course, at this point in the Makeover, you have given up alcohol (and, I would hope, any recreational drugs). Next week, we'll work on smoking, and if you're a smoker, you'll find that this week's suggestions for stress control will help you give up cigarettes.

To combat the effects of stress that cause short- and long-term disease, you must practice a form of relaxation that's active, not passive. Effective relaxation produces demonstrable physiological changes that have been proven to be stress reducing. The goal has to be relaxation itself, not relaxation as a side effect. Real relaxation requires effort and practice. It's not difficult or time consuming, but you have to work at it.

Stress affects your body and your mind. In order to fight stress, it's important to take both into consideration. In working with my patients, I've found that the most effective approach is to relax the body first. I do this by using a modified version of Dr. Herbert Benson's "relaxation response."

Relaxation: The Real Thing

When I searched for a method of relaxation for myself and for my patients that would be simple to learn, relatively fast, and easy to do anywhere, I eventually selected Dr. Herbert Benson's relaxation response as satisfying every criterion. Dr. Benson is a cardiologist associated with Harvard Medical School and Beth Israel Hospital in Boston. Among the first to do extensive research on meditation, he reported on the connection between meditation and reduced blood pressure and the decreased use of drugs. After researching the literature on meditative practices in yoga, Sufism, Zen, Judaism, and Christianity, Dr. Benson distilled the technique, common to all those practices, that produced a quiet mind and a peaceful heart. He called the technique the "relaxation response." It's really a form of demystified meditation.

The relaxation response (RR) is the physiological opposite of the flight-or-fight syndrome generated by stress. It decreases the activity of your sympathetic nervous system as it decreases your metabolism, heart rate, and rate of breathing, decreases the blood flow to your muscles, increases the alpha brainwaves that are associated with feelings of relaxation and well-being, and decreases your blood-lactate levels, which are associated with muscular fatigue. Benson notes that these changes are distinctly different from the physiological changes you experience when you sit quietly or sleep.

Some of my patients initially scoff at the relaxation response. How could something so simple make a difference in the way you feel? Believe me, it does. One patient who was reluctant to do the RR told me, "The truth is, I didn't do the relaxation response for the first few days of my stress week. I thought that once I'd discovered my stress symptoms, knowing them would somehow help me to avoid stress. But of course after a few days I saw this wasn't happening. I tried the relaxation response because everything else on the Makeover had helped me even when I'd been skeptical. After a few days of the RR I felt a noticeable difference. I felt like the master of my ship. At first, I felt that way for a short while after the exercise, but eventually the 'calm time' got longer and longer. In a funny and certainly unexpected way, the stress exercises pulled the whole Makeover together for me. I can't tell you how much better I feel than I did two months ago: I'm calmer, stronger, more energetic, and, I guess best of all, happier."

Here's what you need to invoke the relaxation response:

1. *A Quiet Environment*. This can be anywhere—home or office. Many of my patients sit at their desks and invoke the relaxation response. One man told me that his gym has a "nap room" where people can rest and he uses that. Just be sure to choose a place with no loud noises or distractions.

2. *A Mental Device*. This is equivalent to using a mantra while meditating. It's a single-syllable sound or word that you repeat silently or in a quiet tone. It helps you to remove yourself from logical thought and distractions. Dr. Benson suggests using the word "one." A patient told me she uses the word "snow" in the summer, and "sun" in the winter.

3. *A Passive Attitude*. This sounds simple and it should be, but people sometimes make too much of it, defeating the purpose. A passive attitude means not focusing on how well you're doing in the exercise or whether you're really getting the correct response. When either of these thoughts occurs to you, let it go and focus instead on repeating your chosen word.

4. *A Comfortable Position*. You want to reduce any awareness of your muscles as much as possible. A comfortable chair that supports your head is good. It's even better if you can lie down.

Now here's how you invoke the relaxation response:

1. Sit in a comfortable position in a quiet environment.

2. Close your eyes.

3. Relax your muscles, beginning with your feet, then your calves, thighs, lower torso, chest, shoulders, neck, and head. Pay special attention to the muscles in your neck and face, which tend to get very tense.

4. Breathe through your nose, paying attention to your breathing. As you exhale, say aloud or just think about your chosen word.

5. Do this for at least ten minutes, twenty, if you're able. You can open your eyes to check the time, but Dr. Benson cautions against using an alarm.

For the rest of the Makeover program, make time for the relaxation response twice a day. Think of it as a "mind break" that has taken the place of a coffee break. I think you'll eventually feel that the RR time is the most important part of your day. Patients who practice the relaxation response regularly are always enthusiastic about its calming and invigorating effects.

I find the RR is most effective when done in the middle of the day and then again in the evening. Many of my patients do it just before or after lunch at their desks or at home, or just after work, or before bed at the end of the day. It should become part of your daily routine and it will help you cope with daily stresses in your life on both a physiological and psychological level. You will be amazed to find that such a simple exercise that takes so little time can have such an important effect on your body and mind.

Your Stress Triggers

But what about those stresses that hit like lightning? The driver who cuts in front of you, the plumber who won't return your phone call? These stressful daily incidents that trigger dangerous physiological reactions need immediate action to help mitigate their effects.

The most effective time to combat such stresses is when they occur. But first you must make yourself aware of them.

How do you know when an event is stressful? Often you can tell because you feel anxious. The boss is yelling at you. The baby is sick. But don't count just the obvious stressful events. Here is where you need the list of symptoms on pages 266–268. When you become familiar with these symptoms, you'll be able to pick out the stresses that you may not have suspected were affecting you. For example, your jaws may tighten when you speak to a certain co-worker. You might not count this as stress unless you're alert to your symptoms. Then, when you feel your jaws tighten, you may realize that feelings of competition or resentment make encounters with this colleague stressful.

What's the point of recognizing your stress triggers if you can't change the sources of the stress? It serves two purposes. First it forces you to become aware of what those stressful situations are. You'll probably find that just knowing what stresses you helps you to change your reaction to it. In some instances knowing something stresses you helps you resolve a nagging problem. One of my patients told me she always got a knot in her stomach when her mother called her early in the morning because it meant she would either have to cut her mother short or be late for work. When she realized that the situation was a real problem, she suggested to her mother that she phone in the evening when they would have more time to enjoy a leisurely chat.

Relaxation: A Quick Fix

Now that you recognize your stress triggers, you can learn to deal with them in a positive way. A modification of the relaxation response is the solution I have developed. It works well for me and for my patients. Obviously you can't invoke the relaxation response in the middle of a traffic jam or in a noisy meeting. But if you develop any of the physical symptoms mentioned on page 266 when you encounter these situations, here's a modified relaxation response that will at least help relieve them.

When you notice you're tensing up in a stressful

situation, simply use step 3 of the relaxation response: Consciously relax all your muscles, beginning with your feet and working up to your head. Again, pay special attention to your neck and face muscles. Sometimes when patients demonstrate how they do the relaxation response, they concentrate so hard on doing it right that I can see the muscles twitching in their jaws! Breathe deeply as you do this.

Just this simple technique can help relax you and deflect the wear and tear of stress on your body. Make it a point now to use this technique as often as you can. You'll find that after a period of time it will become almost automatic, and in the long run it can be of real help in fighting stress.

The Stress Advantage

Now you're working to control the effects of stress on your health. This, as I've mentioned, has a corollary benefit: It makes you calmer and more effective in handling everyday affairs. But you can do still more. You can learn to turn stress to your advantage. You do this mainly by working on the way you think about stress.

You've taken the physical approach to relieving stress. Now you're ready to capitalize on stress by altering your state of mind. I have a series of tips gathered from my own experiences and those of my patients. They will help you cope with many aspects of stress. They have one thing in common: They assume that stress is not something you're trying to eliminate from your life. That's an impossible task. Rather, these are tips that will help you face stress as a challenge, an opportunity. You have a choice as to how you react to it. If you can train yourself to view stress as a chance to exert your will and self-control so as to make things happen your way, stress can play a very positive role in your life.

• **FOCUS ON YOUR GOAL:** Many of the most stressful situations that I face, and that my patients tell me about, involve other people—the difficult salesperson, the irrational co-worker, the demanding relative. When we experience these moments, our tendency is to focus on how we feel—enraged, defensive, wounded, diminished, impotent. Unfortunately, by dwelling on these feelings, however justified, we intensify the situation and often wind up escalating the conflict too. Try doing this instead. As soon as you find you are in a potentially stressful situation, try to remove yourself emotionally from it. Forget about what that person did and what you did, and how you have a right to feel a certain way. Instead, ask yourself what you want to happen. How do you want this conflict to be resolved? Once you know what your goal is, you can take action to win that goal.

• **RECOGNIZE** that it's not the major, catastrophic events that are the most dangerous as far as stress is concerned, but the everyday difficulties and how you react to them that will take a toll on you in the long run.

• Try to **ELIMINATE** the words "should" and "must" from conversations with yourself. They represent obligations established by other people. Instead, try to look at your day's activities as challenges to be met and as priorities that you've set for yourself.

• **BE REALISTIC.** Too often we have what seems like a hundred things we want to get done each day, and always feel disappointed in ourselves because we accomplish only a fraction of the list. It's much more efficient and less stressful to set realistic goals.

• Try to do only **ONE THING AT A TIME.** When you catch yourself talking on the phone and reading a letter or working on an unrelated project at a meeting, stop and focus on the task at hand.

• **SET PRIORITIES.** Make a list of what you want to accomplish each day in order of priority. Ignore the bottom of the list; work on the important things first. My busiest and most successful patients have told me that this system works so well that it has not only helped them relieve stress, it has made them far more productive.

• **DE-ESCALATE** your negative emotions. This is a sort of game you play with yourself, but it can be very effective. If you're enraged at someone, decide just to be angry instead. If you feel devastated by some setback, decide just to be disappointed instead.

• **SET GOALS** and work to achieve them. If you can view everyday hassles and tribulations as small problems on the road to a greater goal, you'll have a better perspective on things in general.

• Learn to **SAY NO.** Recognize the fact that you can't always do everything asked of you, and that sometimes other people's requests are distracting you from your goals.

• Learn to **SHARE YOUR CONCERNS** with people close to you. It's remarkable how therapeutic a conversation with a friend or loved one can be when problems are looked at in a fresh light and put into perspective.

• **PAY ATTENTION TO YOUR HEALTH.** If you've reached this point of the Makeover, you're probably in the best of health. Nonetheless, remember that good health—helped by good nutrition and appropriate vitamin supplements—is crucial in avoiding the bad effects of stress.

• **ACCEPT** the fact that you will fail occasionally. When you do, rather than blame yourself, examine the situation with as much distance as you can manage and analyze what you can learn from it.

• **RECOGNIZE** that not everything you do is of crucial importance. If your ego is always on the line, you're shouldering an unreasonable level of stress that will have negative results.

A Note to Nonsmokers

If you don't smoke, congratulations! Not only have you avoided or eliminated one of the worst health risks of our era, you've also completed the Makeover. But I do have a few final words to guide you into the future. So skip this next smokers' week and go on to the final chapter on page 299.

Week Eight: Smoking

Smoking is killing you. It's the single worst habit you could have short of carrying a loaded pistol in your breast pocket. Even worse, you know that it's killing you. It's not like sugar or caffeine—two bad health habits you've already tackled whose damaging effects may have surprised you. Why do you smoke when it's making you feel terrible and shortening your life? Because you're addicted to nicotine. Your body craves it, and every time you try to deprive your body of nicotine, it reacts with outrage, forcing you to light up once again. Nonetheless, this week you're going to stop smoking forever. You're going to break the last and most powerful link in the chain that's keeping you from enjoying total good health.

Your effort to quit smoking is going to be different this time because the Makeover has given you two crucial advantages.

First, you have the psychological advantage of knowing that you can do it. After all, you've already given up sugar, caffeine, and alcohol, improved your nutrition, begun to exercise, and gotten your stress under control. These are major accomplishments. You probably feel more able to quit because you know at first hand what better health really means. And you have the confidence that grows with success. Each bad health habit that you've eliminated has given you increased confidence in your control over your body and in your self-mastery.

You have a physical advantage too. Your body has never been more ready to quit smoking. You won't have to rely entirely on willpower. I believe that if you must count on willpower alone to help you change a habit as ingrained as smoking, your chances of success are not good. But this time when you stop smoking, your body will be working with you instead of against you. I'll explain in a minute how relaxation techniques, vitamin supplements, and control of your blood sugar will all help minimize the effects of nicotine withdrawal and decrease your yearning for a cigarette. As you've improved your overall health, you've actually altered your body's biochemistry. From that standpoint, you're a different person today than you were weeks ago. The new you is physically more ready and able to quit smoking once and for all.

This Week's Goal

This week you're going to stop smoking. You're going to learn why it's crucial to your continued health to make this commitment. You're going to learn why it's been difficult for you to quit in the past and why you will succeed this time. When you've completed the Makeover Seven-Day Plan, you will be cigarette-free.

This week of the Makeover is geared specifically to conquering your physical addiction to nicotine. You'll experience withdrawal, and I'll give you tips that will help you cope with all the symptoms of withdrawal—symptoms that in the past may have sent you right back to lighting up. The key to breaking a physical addiction to nicotine is controlling blood sugar. You've already gotten your blood sugar on an even keel because you've eliminated sugar from your diet and you're taking a chromium supplement. This will make it much easier for you to kick the habit.

Smoking is also a psychological addiction that may take you weeks or even months to conquer because it's so ingrained into your life-style. But once you conquer your physical addiction, which is the hardest part, you'll have the strength to get rid of your psychological addiction. By the end of this week, you will have had your last cigarette, and you will have learned techniques to help you stay away from cigarettes forever. After all, it doesn't count if you only quit for a week. The end of this week is geared to helping you overcome your psychological addiction to cigarettes forever.

What About Weight Gain?

The biggest concern shared by my smoking patients is that if they quit smoking, they'll gain weight. Sometimes they're embarrassed even to mention this because they know that the health benefits of not smoking are so significant that they should be willing to gain a few pounds in order to enjoy these long-term rewards. But I think that any stop-smoking program that ignores possible weight gain is ignoring the real world.

The fact is, though some people who quit smoking maintain a stable weight and some even lose some weight, many people who quit smoking do gain weight. The average weight gain for men is 5.3 pounds. One survey of male smokers revealed that 46 percent who quit smoking for one year gained five pounds or more, 30 percent gained zero to five pounds, and 24 percent actually lost weight or stayed the same.

You're probably familiar with some of the reasons why

ex-smokers gain weight. Snacking instead of smoking is the main problem. The ex-smoker finds that a sharpened sense of taste and smell make food more appealing in addition to giving him something to do with his hands. And some people feel the need to have something in their mouths to replace cigarettes.

Finally there's a connection between the urge to smoke and your blood-sugar level. Smoking can put blood sugar on a roller coaster: Every time you light up, your blood sugar soars, and as the effects of the nicotine wear off, it plummets. This makes you feel tired and weak and edgy. You then yearn for a pick-me-up—a cigarette or perhaps a sweet snack—and the cycle begins again. Unless you cope with this problem, you may find that when you give up cigarettes, you have a powerful urge to eat sweets to keep your blood sugar up. In the Makeover we'll deal directly with the blood-sugar–nicotine connection as well as other incentives to eat.

Some people compalin that they gain weight when they stop smoking even though they swear that they haven't increased their food consumption. Now there's evidence to support their claim. Research has shown that smoking can affect your metabolism. Cigarette smoking stimulates numerous biological functions. For example, oxygen consumption is higher in smokers than in non-smokers. Naturally, if your metabolism is higher when you smoke, and it falls when you stop, you'll gain some weight unless you increase your exercise to compensate. Knowing this, I find that a stepped-up exercise program can help the ex-smoker maintain an optimum weight because, as we know from the exercise week, physical activity actually increases the metabolism.

Because of an improved diet and their exercise programs, most of my patients gain very little extra weight when they quit smoking. Any weight they might gain in the first week or two is usually lost within a couple of months. And even the patients who carry extra pounds for a few months after they quit smoking tell me that it's worth it to be cigarette-free.

Cigarettes and Blood Sugar

The link between nicotine and blood sugar is an important aspect of cigarette addiction. Smoking can actually cause symptoms of hypoglycemia—emotional instability, apprehension, and insecurity. Studies have shown that smoking causes a rapid rise in blood sugar with just as rapid a drop shortly after the cigarette is put out. One Swedish study reported that in some patients the rise in blood sugar was as high as 36 percent. This study concluded that the rapid fall of blood sugar after smoking helps us understand the habit of chain smoking. Once our blood sugar falls, we crave another pick-me-up and reach for another cigarette. We know this uncontrolled rise and fall of the blood-sugar level puts a stress on the body that encourages us to indulge in other unhealthy practices. But by now we have eliminated the worst culprits that encourage the smoking habit: caffeine and sugar.

Knowing the link between blood sugar and nicotine helps our stop-smoking program in two ways: We can avert the need for cigarettes by controlling our blood sugar. We can compensate for the urge to eat sweets by making sure to continue with the chromium supplements we began to take in the sugar week and by working hard to stick with the changes we made in the New Nutrition. I'll have some tips on how to accomplish both these goals later in the chapter.

The Hazards of Smoking

It would be hard to find someone who doesn't know that smoking is dangerous. But most people are unaware of the *range* of dangers that smoking poses to your health.

Smoking is far and away the largest single preventable cause of illness and premature death in the United States. It is associated with heart and blood vessel diseases; chronic bronchitis and emphysema; cancers of the lung, larynx, pharynx, mouth, esophagus, pancreas, and bladder. Smoking has also been connected to other ailments, ranging from minor respiratory infections to stomach ulcers. Smoking during pregnancy increases risks of complications of pregnancy and retarded fetal growth. Tobacco is associated with an estimated 320,000 premature deaths a year. Another ten million Americans currently suffer from debilitating chronic diseases caused by smoking.

Last, but not least, smoking ages you: The Canadian Cancer Society claims that a one-pack-a-day smoker is, at fifty years of age, physically as old as a nonsmoker at fifty-eight.

Not only are you killing yourself by smoking, you're killing those around you. Recent studies on "second-hand smoke" have revealed that the nonsmoking spouse of a smoker has a 23 percent greater chance of developing nicotine-related cancer.

Smokers inhale thousands of chemicals in cigarette smoke, but probably the most dangerous is nitrosamine—the twentieth century's most potent carcinogen. This chemical is found in bacon and cured meats, but one-pack-a-day smokers inhale a hundred times as many nitrosamines as the average American gets from a diet containing cured meats. About twenty-five percent of the other chemicals in tobacco smoke are known to cause cancer, or to cause cancer in association with other chemicals, or to irritate tissues so as to make cancer more likely.

Most people know that it's unwise to have too many X rays taken because of the dangers of radiation. But did you know that a person who smokes one and a half packs of cigarettes a day receives an annual radiation dose equivalent to that of three hundred chest X rays?

Many people feel that even though smoking is dangerous, it's too late, the damage has been done. Here is a chart in which Jane Brody, *New York Times* health columnist, summarizes the American Cancer Society's reasons for "Why You Should Quit Smoking."

WHY YOU SHOULD QUIT SMOKING

Risks of Smoking	*Benefits of Quitting*
Shortened life expectancy Risk proportional to amount smoked. A twenty-five-year-old who smokes two packs a day can expect to live 8.3 years less than nonsmoking contemporary.	After ten to fifteen years, ex-smoker's risk approaches that of those who never smoked.
Lung cancer Cigarettes are major cause in both men and women. Overall, smokers' risk is ten times higher than nonsmokers.	After ten to fifteen years, risk approaches that of those who never smoked.
Larynx cancer Smoking increases risk by 2.9 to 17.7 fold that of nonsmokers.	Gradual reduction in risk, reaching normal after ten years.
Mouth cancer Smokers have three to ten times as many oral cancers as nonsmokers. Alcohol may act as synergist, enhancing effect of smoking.	Reducing or eliminating smoking/drinking lowers risk in first few years. Risk drops to level of nonsmokers in ten to fifteen years.

WHY YOU SHOULD QUIT SMOKING

Risks of Smoking	*Benefits of Quitting*
Cancer of esophagus Smoking increases risk of fatal cancer two to nine times. Alcohol acts as a synergist.	Since risk is proportional to dose, reducing or eliminating smoking/drinking should lower risk.
Cancer of bladder Smokers have seven to ten times greater risk. Synergistic with certain occupational exposures.	Risk decreases gradually to that of nonsmokers over seven years.
Cancer of pancreas Risk of fatal cancer is two to five times higher than for nonsmokers.	Since risk seems related to dose, stopping smoking should reduce it.
Coronary heart disease Smoking a major factor, causing 120,000 excess heart deaths each year.	Risk decreases sharply after one year. After ten years, risk is same as for those who never smoked.
Bronchitis and emphysema Smokers face four to twenty-five times greater risk of death; lung damage even in young smokers.	Cough and sputum disappear within a few weeks. Lung function may improve; deterioration slowed.
Stillbirth and low birth weight Smoking mothers have more stillbirths and babies born at below normal weight, with greater vulnerability to disease and death.	If mother stopped smoking before the fourth month of pregnancy, risk to fetus is eliminated.

WHY YOU SHOULD QUIT SMOKING

Risks of Smoking	Benefits of Quitting
Peptic ulcer Smokers get more ulcers and are more likely to die from them; cure more difficult in smokers.	Ex-smokers get ulcers, too, but they heal faster and more completely than in smokers.
Drug and test effects Smoking changes pharmacological effects of many medicines; changes results of diagnostic tests and increases risk of blood clots from oral contraceptives.	Most blood factors raised by smoking return to normal after quitting. Nonsmokers on birth control pill have much lower risks of hazardous clots and heart attacks.

As you can see, the health hazards of smoking are overwhelming. But it's encouraging to know that they are all almost totally reversible.

Smoking obviously puts your health at severe risk. But it's also responsible for other problems:

• Smoking affects fertility by lowering sperm count and decreasing sperm motility.

• Smoking ages the skin prematurely, causing wrinkles.

• Smoking alters sleep patterns, probably because of the stimulating effect of nicotine. Smokers find it more difficult to get to sleep and more difficult to stay asleep.

• Smoking can cause back pain by decreasing the blood flow to the vertebrae, creating disk problems.

• Smoking makes you and your environment smell.

• Smoking stains your hands and teeth and fouls your breath.

• Smoking is expensive.

Is Cold Turkey Best?

Some people quit by cutting down gradually over a period of weeks or months; some people stop overnight. I have found that a modified cold-turkey method is the most effective.

People who quit cold turkey find that their withdrawal symptoms ease much more quickly than for those who cut down gradually. According to one doctor who works with smokers, if you smoke thirty cigarettes a day—say, one every thirty minutes—you're on the verge of withdrawal about every twenty minutes, which is why you light up as soon as you can. If you decrease your consumption to four cigarettes a day, you're constantly living in withdrawal. But if you quit cold turkey, your body will rid itself of nicotine in about forty-eight hours. Obviously, the sooner you recover from withdrawal, the sooner you'll feel the benefits of not smoking and the easier it will be to avoid cigarettes in the future. But if you live in constant withdrawal, you are never going to lose your craving for nicotine.

The Seven-Day Plan

I have successfully used a seven-day quit-smoking program that is effective and simple to follow. It's worked for others, and it's going to work for you. The method is geared to reduce the amount of nicotine you consume over a period of days, to help you cope with the symptoms of physical withdrawal, and to prepare you for the psychological withdrawal that may linger for weeks or months. In one week you're going to be cigarette-free and feel better than you have in years.

Before You Begin . . .

This is the only week of the Makeover that is affected by what's going on in your life. If you're anticipating a particularly stressful week—if you're going on a difficult business trip, or are in the middle of a divorce or looking for an apartment—this is probably not the best time to stop smoking. It will be too tempting to light up if stress gets to you. I suggest that you wait a week or two before you begin this week of the program.

On the other hand, don't put off this week for more than two or three weeks. It's too easy to procrastinate when facing a challenge like giving up smoking. But if your life is particularly stressful for more than three weeks, it's possible that it is often that way and you could keep smoking forever. In that case, begin this week right away.

Before you begin this week, you must make a serious commitment to stop smoking. If you start with the idea that you'll just "give it a try" without seriously deciding to stop smoking, the effort won't work. But some people find it positively overwhelming to face a lifetime without cigarettes. When patients feel this way, I suggest that they commit themselves to one month without smoking; then they can reevaluate their decision. Usually if they can go a month without smoking, they're eager to quit forever.

I strongly suggest that you begin the smoking week on a Saturday, not while you are on vacation or in any situation that is very different from your regular routine. The reason to start on a Saturday is that your first totally smoke-free day will be on Thursday. It's more effective if people have their smoke-free day near the middle of the week so they don't face a cold-turkey day on the weekend. And it's best to quit smoking while on your regular routine at work or at home, because to do it effectively, you have to learn new behavior patterns and these new patterns must be integrated in your daily life. If you learn to stop smoking while on vacation—swimming and sunning and sailing all day—it will be difficult to avoid cigarettes when you go back to the grind and to all those situations you associate with smoking.

One final word: Some of the things that you must do in this week's program may sound gimmicky. Making a list on the first day, for example, may seem like something you might just as well skip, as it's not going to affect your decision to quit. Please realize that there's a reason for all the suggestions in the program. Some are optional and are noted as such. But the others should be taken seriously if you expect to succeed. Remember, it's only one week and the rewards will be worth it.

Day One

Today's goal is to make the commitment to quit smoking and to build motivation to stick with that commitment. You're not going to make any effort actually to stop smoking today, so smoke as many cigarettes as you ordinarily would.

• **MAKE A LIST** of all the reasons why you want to stop smoking. The list could include health reasons, but also very personal and practical reasons. One of my patients said that a compelling motivation was to rid her apartment of the smell of tobacco. One brisk autumn day, after a walk in the park, she came home with a friend and was embarrassed to notice for the first time how stale and smoky her apartment smelled. Other reasons might include the cost of smoking, getting rid of smoker's cough, freeing yourself of paraphernalia like lighters and ashtrays, improving your ability to taste and smell, improving your lung capacity for exercise, and so forth.

• **MARK DAY SIX ON YOUR CALENDAR.** It will be your first smoke-free day.

• **ENLIST HELPERS.** If you can get someone to stop smoking with you, so much the better. A spouse or a friend who is serious about it can be a valuable ally. But don't ask people to quit with you who aren't really committed; they may backslide and take you with them. Also be wary of spouses and other people who belittle your efforts or won't support you. I've known of smoking spouses who've undermined the efforts of a husband or wife to kick the habit. Sometimes smoking is an activity that two people share in very pleasurable moments of their lives and the smoker is reluctant to see the other person give it up. Be understanding of these feelings if you encounter them, but be firm in your conviction that you are determined to stop smoking.

• **MAKE A BUTT JAR.** This is a jar that's big enough to hold about a day's worth of cigarette butts. It's best if it's small enough to carry around with you, and it should have a lid. As you go through the day, fill the jar with cigarette butts. If you find yourself wavering in your commitment to quit, take a whiff of your butt jar.

• **REVIEW THE NEW NUTRITION** in Week Three of the Makeover. It's important to make a special point of sticking with the principles of the New Nutrition when you stop smoking, since a good diet will help you cope with any withdrawal symptoms you might experience as you go through the week.

Day Two

Today you're going to figure out what prompts you to smoke. You'll still be smoking as much as you want, but you'll be paying attention to when and how much you smoke.

• **SWITCH CIGARETTE BRANDS.** Most of my patients find it effective to switch to a mentholated brand if they smoke regular cigarettes, and vice versa.

• No matter how much you smoke, **BUY ONLY ONE PACK OF CIGARETTES AT A TIME.**

• **MAKE A "SMOKING TRIGGER" LIST.** Take a small piece of paper and wrap it around your cigarette pack with a rubber band. Each time you light up a ciagrette, make a note of the time and what you are doing. For example, you might note you have a cigarette at 9:30 A.M. while you're on the phone, or a cigarette at 1:00 P.M. after lunch, or a cigarette at 3:00 P.M. while you're working on a project or while driving, and so forth. The point is to make you aware of the circumstances that stimulate you to light up. Some people smoke unconsciously—they simply light up regularly. Other people smoke mainly for pleasure—say, with a cup of coffee or after a meal. Still others smoke when they are working or when they are nervous or bored. Your list will help you to discover what prompts you to smoke. It will also make you focus on the act of smoking itself; you won't be lighting up unconsciously because you have to make a note when you smoke each cigarette.

Day Three

Today you're going to begin to cut down on your smoking.

• **REVIEW YOUR LIST OF REASONS FOR QUITTING** and see if you can add any more. Think about the feelings of satisfaction and self-control you'll have when you stop.

• **STUDY YOUR TRIGGER LIST** to see if there are any times of day or occasions on which you smoke which you can eliminate. It's usually most effective to eliminate the cigarettes that don't mean as much to you. For example, you may really take pleasure in your cigarette after dinner, but not mind so much eliminating one smoked in midmorning.

• **TRY TO ELIMINATE ONE QUARTER OF YOUR USUAL DAILY NUMBER OF CIGARETTES.**

• Every time you feel as if you want a cigarette, **WAIT TEN MINUTES BEFORE YOU LIGHT UP.**

• **ADD BUTTS TO YOUR BUTT JAR,** if it isn't full already, and put an inch or so of water in the bottom. Make a point of smelling the contents occasionally. That's what your clothes, your furniture, the inside of your car, etc., smell like when you smoke.

• **BE SURE TO TAKE CHROMIUM.** Review Week Two on sugar, and make every effort to keep your blood sugar on an even keel. Don't forget to take your chromium. As you cut down on cigarettes, you may begin to experience symptoms of withdrawal. If your blood sugar is under control, these symptoms will be lessened and your task will be much easier.

Day Four

Today you're going to gain more confidence and self-control by further cutting down your daily consumption of cigarettes.

• **REVIEW YOUR REASONS FOR QUITTING.** It's best to do this first thing in the morning.

• **CUT DOWN ON CIGARETTES SMOKED** by reviewing your trigger list and choosing certain situations in which you won't smoke. For example, decide not to smoke at all while talking on the phone or while driving.

• **PRACTICE "PSEUDOSMOKING":** When you feel the desire for a cigarette, purse your lips and inhale through your mouth. Hold your breath for a minute and blow it out through your mouth. This can not only satisfy your urge for a cigarette, but the deep breathing will relax you and make it easier to hold to your conviction to quit.

• When you feel an urge to smoke, **DELAY FIFTEEN MINUTES** before lighting up.

• While you're smoking, **PUT YOUR CIGARETTE**

DOWN BETWEEN PUFFS. Try to wait a full minute between puffs.

• **DON'T CARRY A LIGHTER OR MATCHES** around with you, so each time you want to have a cigarette you must ask someone for a light.

Day Five

This is your last day of smoking. Today you're going to continue to cut down on your cigarette consumption, learn to find substitutes, and announce your plans to quit to friends and co-workers.

• **REVIEW YOUR LIST OF REASONS TO QUIT** first thing in the morning. Take a minute to recognize the progress you've already made: You've cut down on smoking, and by this time tomorrow you will be an ex-smoker.

• **ANNOUNCE TO FRIENDS AND CO-WORKERS** that tomorrow you're going to stop smoking.

• **TRY TO SMOKE HALF THE NUMBER OF CIG-ARETTES** you smoked on the first day of the program.

• **USE THE WRONG HAND TO SMOKE WITH** so that the act of smoking becomes awkward.

• **FIND TACTILE SUBSTITUTES FOR SMOKING.** Worry beads are popular with my patients. You can still find them in some Indian import stores. Keep them in your pocket and reach for them whenever you feel the urge to smoke. You can also try a plastic cigarette. I know that these things may sound gimmicky, but remember that you'll only be using them as a temporary crutch to get through the first week.

• **FIND ORAL SUBSTITUTES FOR SMOKING.** Buy some sugarless or low-calorie snacks. Eat sugarless gum or candy (this is the only time I recommend you indulge in artificially sweetened candy), celery sticks, or any other nutritious low-calorie snacks you enjoy.

Day Six

This is your first smoke-free day.

• **REVIEW YOUR REASONS FOR QUITTING.** Do this first thing in the morning. Spend a minute renewing your commitment to stop smoking.

• **REVIEW THE SYMPTOMS OF WITHDRAWAL** in the next section of this book so you'll know what to expect.

• **USE ALL OF YOUR SUBSTITUTES AND DISTRACTIONS.** Use your worry beads or plastic cigarette. Eat your low-calorie or sugarless snacks.

• **TAKE A SHOWER OR BATH.** It will help relax you.

• **THROW OUT ANY REMAINING CIGARETTES OR SMOKING PARAPHERNALIA.** Don't just toss cigarettes into the trash can. Wet them first so you couldn't possibly be tempted.

• **USE YOUR BUTT JAR.** Sniff it whenever you feel like having a cigarette.

• **INCREASE YOUR EXERCISE.** Lengthen your exercise session by ten or fifteen minutes. The increased activity will help you combat any withdrawal symptoms, including increased fatigue, tingling in the arms and legs, and reduced metabolism caused by the nicotine leaving your body.

Day Seven

You've gotten through one smoke-free day and you're going to do it again. Today you'll need to reaffirm your commitment to being a nonsmoker.

• **REVIEW YOUR REASONS FOR QUITTING** first thing in the morning. You should be proud of having gotten through one day without smoking: You're well on your way to your goal.

• **INCREASE THE RELAXATION EXERCISES** you

learned last week. Tension, anxiety, anger—almost any kind of stress—will make you yearn for a cigarette. Head these feelings off by doing your relaxation exercises.

• **DRINK PLENTY OF FRUIT JUICES.** The natural sugar in fruit juices will give your blood sugar a boost and will slow the effects of nicotine withdrawal on your body. Some people claim that orange juice and tómato juice are best.

• **USE YOUR BUTT JAR.** Sniff it whenever you feel the urge for a cigarette.

• **PLAN A WEEKEND ACTIVITY THAT WILL PUT YOU IN A NONSMOKING SITUATION.** Visit a museum or see a play. Make an effort to engage in a pleasurable activity for your first nonsmoking weekend. It's important that you keep busy and best if you do so with nonsmoking friends.

• **REWARD YOURSELF.** You've been through a difficult week. Treat yourself to a weekend at an inn or some new clothes or dinner at an elegant restaurant. One of my patients figured out how much money she would be saving in a year of not smoking, and she spent a day at the racetrack betting those savings.

Withdrawal: What to Expect

Some people stop smoking and have no symptoms whatsoever. They're the lucky ones. Most people notice some symptoms. For certain people, the symptoms are mild, while for others, withdrawal is terribly difficult. Here's a rundown of what you might experience when you quit smoking:

• **CRAVING:** You will most likely feel a physical desire for a cigarette. Fortunately, if you've been through the Makeover, the craving should be minimized because your blood sugar is under control and you're taking chromium supplements to help stabilize it. Craving is the most difficult aspect for most people. Sometimes the desire for a cigarette can last long after you have had your final one. Look at the "Some Tips from Quitters" on page 297 to help you deal with the craving.

• **HEADACHES:** Some people find that when they stop smoking they suffer temporarily from headaches. Though the reasons why an ex-smoker should develop headaches are unknown, the American Lung Association has suggested remedies: extra rest, deep breathing, and increased exercise. If you develop headaches, be sure to avoid pain relievers that contain caffeine. If you take these, you can put yourself back on a blood-sugar roller coaster and only exacerbate your headaches.

• **COUGH:** When you smoke, this paralyzes the hairlike structures that clean the lungs by sweeping out foreign material. When you stop smoking, these structures regain their function and work overtime to clear the lungs of tar. The ex-smoker's cough is a temporary symptom, and I suggest you let it run its course.

• **TINGLING OR NUMBNESS:** You may have these feelings in your arms or legs. They indicate that you're regaining the optimum circulation that was impaired by smoking. Eventually the sensations will disappear.

• **NERVOUSNESS AND TENSION:** These are common complaints, directly related to the withdrawal of nicotine from your system. The best antidote is to eat lots of fruit which help slow nicotine's release from the body and thereby ease your symptoms. Exercise can be very helpful as a tension reliever for the ex-smoker.

• **TIREDNESS:** As we know, nicotine causes the body to release the antistress hormones that stimulate a state of arousal. The person who is used to this sensation may well feel tired when the artificial stimulation is withdrawn. The remedy is to exercise a bit more than usual and get plenty of rest—some of my patients report that an extra hour of sleep per night for a week or two is a help.

• **LACK OF CONCENTRATION AND DIZZINESS:**
When you smoked, your brain was being deprived of a
certain amount of oxygen. When you stop smoking, the
increased oxygen you're getting can cause these symptoms. Within a few days, you'll become adjusted to this
and the symptoms will disappear.

• **SORE THROAT:** Tobacco numbs the throat. When
you stop smoking, your throat regains full sensation and
begins to recover from the damage smoking has done.
This sore throat will disappear in a week or two. In the
meantime, some patients report that sucking on sugarless
candy helps ease the irritation.

• **CONSTIPATION:** Nicotine is a stimulant and it
works on your bowel function. When you stop smoking,
you may find that your system is sluggish, though most of
my patients suffer minimal constipation because of the
increased fiber they've been eating. If you have trouble
with constipation, review the New Nutrition chapter,
looking especially for ways to increase your fiber intake.

Some Tips from Quitters

I've never smoked, but some of my patients have
passed on tips that they've found helpful in their fight
against tobacco. Here they are:

• Always try to sit in the nonsmoking section of a plane
or restaurant. Try to get a seat far from the smoking
section, as you don't want to have to breathe someone
else's tobacco smoke. This holds particularly true if you're
nervous about flying.

• Don't allow yourself to get hungry. If you do, you'll
find that your blood sugar drops and your resolve weakens. Using the New Nutrition guidelines, eat regular
meals and be sure to have low-calorie snacks on hand at
all times.

• Always have something around to keep your hands

occupied. One patient told me he always carried tooth-picks with him and chewed them constantly.

• Get your clothes, curtains, upholstery, etc., cleaned to rid them of the smell of tobacco. One woman patient told me that not only was it satisfying to have an apartment free of the smell of smoke, the money she had invested in cleaning it kept her from lighting up again.

• When you have the urge to smoke, wash your hands. This replaces one behavior with another, and it can be very effective.

• Try to avoid situations that involve heavy smoking—at least for your first smoke-free month. These events might include card games, cocktail parties, etc.

• One patient told me that when he feels an over-powering urge to smoke, he lights a match, takes a deep breath, blows it out, and crushes it in an ashtray.

• Remember that one cigarette *does* hurt: If you never have "just one cigarette," you won't have to worry about having another and another...

• Remember to take one day at a time. If you do backslide, don't decide you've failed. Just get out your list of reasons for quitting and read through this chapter again. Remember that no one ever died from stopping, but millions have died from smoking.

Your Madeover Future

Makeover Momentum

Congratulations! You've fulfilled the most important commitment you'll ever make. You've dramatically changed your "vital statistics." By eliminating from your life-style the major causes of disease and death in our time, you've increased your chances of a longer, more vigorous life. And, as you now know, you don't have to wait for years to reap the benefits of the changes you've made: You already feel better than you have in years. You're stronger, calmer, more energetic and optimistic than ever before. And probably the biggest surprise was how easy it was to do. Your body has become your ally. You've learned that you don't have to struggle to be healthy.

If you're like many of my patients, you probably began the Makeover with a certain amount of skepticism. Why should this plan work when others haven't? How will you be able to stick to it even if it does work? How many times have I heard patients tell me, "I'll try it, but when it's over I'm going back to business as usual!" It never troubles me when people say this because I have yet to find anyone who has completed the Makeover and still yearns to go back to his or her old ways. I know that if they can get through the eight weeks, they'll be hooked. Now that you've been through the eight weeks, you know why. You just feel too good to go back to the old days. You've discovered the Makeover momentum that carries you into a whole new phase of your life.

There will be times when you may revert. Maggie P., a mother with two children who does free-lance illustrating, told me about her experience:

"I had finished the Makeover and was feeling great. A few months went by and I had no trouble sticking to all the changes I'd made. In fact, it had really become a new way of life for me. Then an old friend from college visited. She was with me for a weekend, and I reverted to every bad habit I'd ever had except for smoking—I knew that I couldn't start that again. But I stayed up late, drank a lot of wine in the evening, ate junk foods—things I hadn't eaten since college—and spent two long mornings drinking coffee with her and catching up on old times. She left Sunday night. Monday morning was horrible. I woke up feeling terrible. I was in a bad mood, was exhausted and irritable. It was a real slap in the face. I realized I hadn't felt that way since I'd begun the Makeover. It really brought home to me how much I'd changed and how much it meant to me to feel good. I got right back on track and have been there ever since."

In a less dramatic way, I notice the Makeover momentum myself on occasional weekends. Whenever I have too much wine—which might be three glasses—I wake up the next morning feeling tired and dragged out. It amazes me every time: It's so easy to convince yourself that just a few glasses of wine won't make much difference. But they do! And I'm glad they do because it reminds me of how I used to feel, and how important it is to feel good now, every single day. And it makes it easy to stick to the principles of the Makeover.

Makeover Missteps

The Makeover has changed your life, but you're still human. The last thing I want to encourage is Makeover fanatics, and I know that the day will come when you'll indulge in a drink or a piece of cake. I think that when this happens, it won't be because you feel a need for these things, but rather because you're in a situation—probably a social one—where it seems almost rude to abstain. At least, that's been my experience and that of my patients. When this happens, there's one important thing to remember:

Don't think because you don't feel awful immediately that it's ok to adopt one of your old bad habits. One piece of cake or one drink may seem to have very little effect on you. This is deceptive. The worse effect may be no effect at all, because it makes you believe that you can continue to indulge. Before you know it, you're back to a pastry-and-coffee break, and you won't feel well. But because your backsliding happened over a period of weeks, you never connected it to undoing your Makeover.

Allow yourself the occasional indulgence. But recognize it as an act that is damaging your health and jeopardizing that great feeling you've been having, and don't repeat it.

What Now?

Here's some advice on how to carry the achievements of the Makeover into the future:

Caffeine
Now that you've finished the Makeover, I know I don't have to urge you to avoid caffeine forever. For one thing, it's easy to do. For another, I'm sure you don't miss it at all. And finally, if you do find yourself in a situation

where you drink a cup of coffee, the aftereffects—feeling very edgy and anxious—will be all the convincing you'll need never to do it again. You may develop a headache. You'll notice a sudden energy drop a few hours after you ingest the caffeine, and you probably won't sleep well that night. Every patient who has had an encounter with caffeine after completion of the Makeover has reported that the aftereffects were dramatic—certainly enough to keep him or her from making the same mistake again.

Sugar

Sugar, like caffeine, is usually happily avoided by Makeover veterans. After banishing sugar for the duration of the Makeover, you'll probably find that your taste has become more sophisticated: Sweet things seem cloying and unappealing. This is usually enough to help keep you away from sugar. You'll also find that you don't have the energy drops that used to make a doughnut or a candy bar seem so tempting. Your stabilized blood sugar has, in effect, strengthened your willpower. I tell my patients that they should continue to avoid sugar completely. But an occasional sweet—and by occasional I mean once every two or three months—is not going to do great damage. You certainly can have a piece of wedding cake or sample a dessert in a three-star Parisian restaurant without doing much harm. But again, you'll probably feel little desire for sweets and will need only one bite of a sugary dessert to confirm this.

Nutrition

The changes you've made in your everyday nutrition should continue for the rest of your life. This New Nutrition is the core of your Makeover. It won't be difficult to continue with it because it quickly becomes a way of life for Makeover veterans.

Vitamins and Minerals

Of course, you'll continue with your regimen of vitamins and minerals. But by the time you've completed the Makeover, you may need to modify the dosages. For example, if you were taking vitamins to compensate for smoking, you can discontinue them now. I suggest that you go back to the vitamin and mineral week and answer the vitamin-mineral questionnaire again. Modify your supplements accordingly.

Alcohol

I've found that alcohol is the secret danger in the future of many people's Makeover. I don't think it's crucial to avoid alcohol completely for the rest of your life UNLESS you're the sort of person who will never be able to have an occasional drink without falling into a pattern of drinking too much. In the alcohol week, I talked about the new "problem" drinkers. These are people who follow a pattern of gradually increasing levels of alcohol consumption. It you recognize yourself in this group, then you should avoid alcohol completely. And, of course, if you have no desire for alcohol, you should avoid it completely. But if you think you can, it's possible to have an occasional drink without undoing the good of the Makeover. I find I can drink one or two glasses of wine on a weekend without ill effects. I definitely notice the difference in the way I feel in the morning, but it's not dramatic enough to be troubling. On the other hand, on the few occasions when I've had two or three glasses of wine at night, I've paid the price the next morning with fatigue, sluggishness, and a headache. Many of my patients report similar reactions. If you do decide to have an occasional drink, limit yourself to one or two per week and NEVER go over that limit. If you suddenly find you are having a drink almost every night, repeat Week Five of the Makeover. Remember that the danger from alcohol—

from the point of view of the Makeover—is increasing your tolerance. You want to avoid this at all costs.

Exercise

Exercise is now a permanent part of your life. You may become even more interested in it as you begin to enjoy its many benefits. As I mentioned earlier, when I began to compete in triathlons, I got more and more enthusiastic about the good effects of exercise on my mind and body. But even if you just continue with a regular program of walking, you'll be so conscious of how great it makes you feel that by the time you've completed the Makeover, you'll be an exercise convert. Remember, too, that exercise, like stress control, is a sort of catalyst for all the good effects of the Makeover. If you continue with all your other Makeover achievements but skip exercise, you'll feel good—but not great.

Stress Control

Even though you've been working on stress control for only a week (if you were a nonsmoker) or two (if you were a smoker,) you already know how important it is. You should continue with your relaxation-response exercises for the rest of your life. The benefits are cumulative. While last week you may have only just been able to clear your mind, this week you're finding that you can draw on increasing reserves of mental energy as you practice your daily relaxation exercises. Over time your ability to focus your energies will increase as will your self-mastery and sense of purpose.

Smoking

You will never smoke again.

I think that you'll find the changed metabolism and increased strength and willpower that you enjoy as a result of the Makeover will make it easy to avoid smoking for the rest of your life. It's absolutely crucial that you do so. Some people lose their yearning for a cigarette quickly—in a week or two. For others, it's a struggle that takes months. Some patients find that the idea of smoking a cigarette never loses its appeal. But they still manage to stay nonsmokers. The trick is constant reaffirmation of your desire to be a nonsmoker. You may find that you need to read the material in the smoking week regularly to boost your resolve. You may also find that reading the other books containing stop-smoking programs are helpful. Read these books *before* you weaken and have a smoke. Read them whenever you feel your determination faltering. At least one good effect of quitting smoking is felt immediately: Your body has already begun to recover from the damaging effects of smoking on your health. In time, you will have almost completely reduced your risk of nicotine-linked disease.

Most of my patients live happily ever after without another cigarette. One woman wrote to tell me that after the Makeover, during which she quit a fifteen-year habit, she couldn't figure out why she had ever smoked at all. I'm really convinced that if you stick with the changes you've made throughout the Makeover, your improved metabolism, your strengthened willpower, and your heightened sense of self-mastery will make you an ex-smoker forever.

A New Beginning

I hope that for you, as for my patients, the Makeover has become a new beginning. You no longer take your health for granted. You're no longer willing to settle for sluggish mornings and tired afternoons. My patients tell me that this new awareness of how they feel has been the most important overall change in their lives since the Makeover. They've gained a fine-tuned appreciation of the state of their health. Not that they've become obsessive, but now they know how they should feel, how they want to feel.

A friend, who is a veteran of the Makeover, told me that the Makeover was a sort of renaissance for him. "I used to ignore how I felt unless I was so sick that I couldn't work. Now I take pleasure every day in how I feel. When I wake up with energy and enthusiasm, I notice it because I know that there was a time when it took me almost until lunch to wake up. I feel like a new person, and though I really like the idea that I'm healthier and look better, what I like the most is that I feel like a new person—I'm optimistic and energetic. I like the new me."

I hope that you think of the Makeover as a new beginning. I hope that you don't think of yourself as having finished something, but rather as having begun a whole new phase of your life—one that will be more rewarding than the phase you've completed. Because, in fact, you have been made over, and the new you is something special—a really healthy person.

New Confidence

You're well aware of how the Makeover has made you feel physically. But there's a spillover benefit that you're probably also experiencing. Most of my patients report that one of the unexpected pleasures of the Makeover is the boost it gives to their self-confidence. Why? I think it's a combination of things. First of all, you look better and that always makes you feel good. You've probably lost weight. Your body is probably firmer than it has been in years. You skin and eyes are clearer than ever. You have a vibrant look that only good health can produce.

You also have an exhilarating feeling of self-mastery. You are in control. All those diets that failed, those exercise routines left by the wayside, those good resolutions quickly abandoned are ghosts of the past. This time you're a success. This time you've really changed your life, and it feels good.

One patient told me that she values this feeling more than any other benefit of the Makeover. "I look great and I have tons of energy. But best of all, I proved that I could do it and, believe me, two months ago I was a lost cause. It would be embarrassing to tell you the number of self-improvement programs I've abandoned. But this one worked. I had some weak moments, but I did it. It's affected every aspect of my life. If I can do this, I can do anything."

This new confidence can be even more valuable than improved health because it's confidence that will help you keep on track, enjoying the benefits of the Makeover for years to come.

Again, congratulations. You've done something extraordinary: You've changed your life. But the adventure is just beginning. Make the best of it. Nothing can stop you now.

Sources

PART I

Archart-Treichel, Joan. *Biotypes: The Critical Link Between Your Personality and Your Health*. New York: Times Books, 1980.

Benson, Herbert. *The Mind/Body Effect*. New York: Simon & Schuster, 1979.

Bloomfield, Harold, and Robert Kory. *The Holistic Way to Health and Happiness*. New York: Simon & Schuster, 1978.

Cousins, Norman. *The Healing Heart*. New York: W. W. Norton & Company, 1983.

Davidson, Park O., and Sheena M. Davidson, eds. *Behavioral Medicine: Changing Health Lifestyles*. New York: Brunner/Mazel, 1980.

Davis, Joel. *Endorphins: New Waves in Brain Chemistry*. New York: Dial Press, 1984.

Farquhar, John, M.D. *The American Way of Life Need Not Be Hazardous to Your Health*. New York: W. W. Norton, 1978.

Flynn, Patricia. *Holistic Health*. Englewood Cliffs, N.J.: Prentice-Hall, 1980.

Harris, Louis. *Healthy Lifestyles, Unhealthy Lifestyles*. New York: Garland Publishing, 1984.

Hatterer, Lawrence J. *The Pleasure Addicts*. New York: A. S. Barnes & Company, 1980.

Keefe, Francis J., and James A. Blumenthal. *Assessment Strategies in Behavioral Medicine*. New York: Grune & Stratton, 1982.

Lewy, Robert, M.D. *Preventive Primary Medicine*. Boston: Little Brown & Company, 1980.

Palm, Daniel J. *Diet Away Your Stress, Tension and Anxiety*. New York: Doubleday & Company, 1976.

Pelletier, Kenneth R. *Holistic Medicine*. New York: Delacorte Press, 1979.

Pinkerton, Susan, Howard Hughes, and W. W. Wenrich. *Behavioral Medicine: Clinical Applications*. New York: John Wiley & Sons, 1982.

Selye, Hans. *Stress Without Distress*. New York: J. B. Lippincott Company, 1974.

————. *The Stress of Life*. New York: McGraw-Hill Book Company, 1978.

U.S. Department of Health, Education and Welfare. *Healthy People: The Surgeon General's Report on Health Promotion and Disease Prevention*. Washington D.C., 1979.

PART II

Week One: Caffeine

Brody, Jane. *Jane Brody's Nutrition Book*. New York: W. W. Norton & Company, 1981.

Goulart, Frances Sheridan. *The Caffeine Book*. New York: Dodd, Mead & Company, 1984.

Massey, Robert, and J. K. Wise. "Effects of Caffeine on Urinary Excretion of Minerals." *Nutrition Research*, 4(1):43–50, January/February 1984.

Morck, et al. "Tea, Coffee and Iron Absorption." *American Journal of Clinical Nutrition*, 37(3):416–420, 1983.

Palm, Daniel J. *Diet Away Your Stress, Tension and Anxiety*. New York: Doubleday & Company, 1976.

Saifer, Phyllis, M.D., and Merla Zellerback. *Detox*. Los Angeles: Jeremy P. Tarcher, 1984.

Spindel, Wurtman, McCall, et al. "Neuroendocrine Effects of Caffeine in Normal Subjects." *Clinical Pharmaceutical Therapy*, September 1984, pp. 402–407.

Weil, Andrew, and Winifrcd Rosen. *Chocolate to Morphine: Understanding Mind-Active Drugs*. Boston: Houghton Mifflin & Company, 1983.

Week Two: Sugar

Bland, Jeffrey. *Your Health Under Siege: Using Nutrition to Fight Back*. Brattleboro, Vt.: Stephen Greene Press, 1981.

―――. *Nutraerobics*. San Francisco: Harper & Row, 1983.

Cannon, Geoffrey, and Hetty Einzig. *Dieting Makes You Fat*. New York: Simon & Schuster, 1983.

Food and Nutrition Board, National Academy of Sciences. "Recommended Dietary Allowances," 9th ed. Washington, D.C.: U.S. Government Printing Office, 1980.

Jeejeebhoy, A. N., R. C. Chu, and A. Bruce-Robinson. "Chromium Deficiency, Glucose Intolerance, and Neuropathy Reversed by Chromium Supplementation." *American Journal of Clinical Nutrition*, June 30 (1977), pp. 531–539.

Johnson, D., K. E. Dorr, W. M. Swenson, and J. Service. "Reactive Hypoglycemia." *Journal of the American Medical Association*, March 21, 1980, pp. 1151–1155.

Leichter, S. "Alimentary Hypoglycemia: A New Appraisal." *American Journal of Clinical Nutrition* 41 (October 1979), pp. 2104–2114.

Lewy, Robert. *Preventive Primary Medicine*. Boston: Little Brown & Company, 1980.

Null, Gary. *The Complete Guide to Health and Nutrition*. New York: Delacorte Press, 1984.

Palm, Daniel J. *Diet Away Your Stress, Tension and Anxiety*. New York: Doubleday & Company, 1976.

Saunders, Jeraldine, and Harvey Ross. *Hypoglycemia: The Disease Your Doctor Won't Treat*. New York: Pinnacle Books, 1980.

Week Three: Nutrition Improvement

Bland, Jeffrey. *Your Health Under Siege: Using Nutrition to Fight Back*. Brattleboro, Vt.: Stephen Greene Press. 1981.

Brewster, Letitia, and Michael Jacobson. *The Changing American Diet*. Washington, D.C.: Center for Science in the Public Interest, 1978.

Brody, Jane. *Jane Brody's Nutrition Book*. New York: W. W. Norton & Company, 1980.

Cannon, Geoffrey, and Hetty Einzig. *Dieting Makes You Fat*. New York: Simon & Schuster, 1983.

Einsberger, John. "Death of Dieting." *American Health Magazine*, January/February, 1985, p. 29.

Farquhar, John W., M.D. *The American Way of Life Need Not Be Hazardous to Your Health*. New York: W. W. Norton & Company, 1978.

Goulart, Frances Sheridan. *Nutritional Self-Defense*. New York: Dodd, Mead & Company, 1984.

Levenson, Frederick. *The Causes and Prevention of Cancer*. New York: Stein & Day, 1985.

Nash, Joyce, and Linda Ormiston. *Taking Charge of Your Weight and Well-Being*. Palo Alto, Calif.: Bull Publishing Company, 1978.

Null, Gary. *The Complete Guide to Health and Nutrition*. New York: Delacorte Press, 1984.

Pritikin, Nathan. *The Pritikin Promise*. New York: Simon & Schuster, 1983.

Scrimshaw, N., and V. Young. "The Requirements of Human Nutrition." *Scientific American,* August 1973, pp. 51–64.

Williams, R. *Nutrition Against Disease.* New York: Bantam Books, 1973.

Wright, Jonathan V. *Dr. Wright's Book of Nutritional Therapy.* Emmaus, Pa.: Rodale Press, 1979.

Week Four: Vitamins and Minerals, the New Nutrition Supplements

Benowicz, Robert J. *Vitamins and You.* New York: Berkley Books, 1981.

Bland, Jeffrey. *Your Health Under Siege: Using Nutrition to Fight Back.* Brattleboro, Vt.: Stephen Greene Press, 1981.

———. *Nutraerobics.* San Francisco: Harper & Row, 1983.

Bloomfield, Harold, and Robert Kory. *The Holistic Way to Health and Happiness.* New York: Simon & Schuster, 1978.

Brody, Jane. *Jane Brody's Nutrition Book.* New York: W. W. Norton & Company, 1981.

Editors of *Prevention. Vitamins for Better Health.* Emmaus, Pa.: Rodale Press, 1982.

Food and Nutrition Board, National Academy of Sciences. "Recommended Dietary Allowances," 9th ed. Washington, D.C.: U.S. Government Printing Office, 1980.

Hendler, Sheldon Saul, M.D. *The Complete Guide to Anti-Aging Nutrients.* New York: Simon & Schuster, 1985.

Kirschmann, John D., with Lavon J. Dunne. *Nutrition Almanac.* New York: McGraw-Hill Book Company, 1984.

Pangborn, T., and R. Hamilton. "Vitamin E Content of Home Prepared Versus Commercially Prepared Entrees." *Journal of the American Dietetics Association*, June 1976.

Rosenberg, Harold. *The Doctor's Book of Vitamin Therapy*. New York: G. P. Putnam's Sons, 1974.

Williams, Roger. *Biochemical Individuality: The Basis of the Genetotropic Concept*. New York: John Wiley & Sons, 1956.

———. *Nutrition Against Disease*. New York: Bantam Books, 1973.

———, and Dwight Kalita, eds. A *Physician's Handbook on Orthomolecular Medicine*. New Canaan, Conn.: Keats, 1980.

Week Five: Alcohol

Brody, Jane. *Jane Brody's Nutrition Book*. New York: W. W. Norton & Company, 1981.

Farquhar, John. *The American Way of Life Need Not Be Hazardous to Your Health*. New York: W. W. Norton. 1978.

Palm, Daniel J. *Diet Away Your Stress, Tension and Anxiety*. New York: Doubleday & Company, 1976.

Saifer, Phyllis, M.D., and Merla Zellerback. *Detox*. Los Angeles: Jeremy P. Tarcher, 1984.

Vogler, Roger, M.D., and Wayne Bartz, M.D. *The Better Way to Drink*. New York: Simon & Schuster, 1982.

Weil, Andrew, and Winifred Rosen. *Chocolate to Morphine: Understanding Mind-Active Drugs*. Boston: Houghton Mifflin, 1983.

Week Six: Exercise

Brody, Jane. *Personal Health*. New York: Times Books, 1982.

Cooper, Ken. *Aerobics*. New York: Bantam Books, 1968.

Diethrich, Edward B., M.D. *The Arizona Heart Institute's Heart Test*. New York: Simon & Schuster, 1981.

Hales, Dianne, and Robert E. Hales, M.D. *The U.S.*

Army Total Fitness Program. New York: Crown Publishers, 1985.

Harris, T. George. "The End of the Diet Era." *American Health,* May 1985, p. 48.

Jonas, Margaret, and David Silver. "The Last Cure All." *American Health,* May 1985, p. 62.

Katch, F. I., and William D. McArdle. *Nutrition, Weight Control and Exercise*. Boston: Houghton Mifflin, 1977.

Leon, A. S., J. Conrad, and D. Hunninghake. "Effects of Vigorous Walking on Body Composition, and Carbohydrate and Lipid Metabolism of Obese Young Men." *Medical Journal of Clinical Nutrition,* September 1979, pp. 1776–1787.

Mirkin, Gabe, and Marshall Hoffman. *The Sportsmedicine Book*. New York: Little Brown & Company, 1978.

Rosenzweig, Sandra. *Sportsfitness for Women*. New York: Harper & Row, 1982.

Week Seven: Stress Control

Benson, H., J. D. Beary, and M. P. Carol. "The Relaxation Response." *Psychiatry* (37), 37–46. 1974.

Brody, Jane. *Personal Health*. New York: Times Books, 1982.

Cousins, Norman. *The Healing Heart*. New York: W. W. Norton & Company, 1983.

LeShan, L. "Psychological States as Factors in the Development of Malignant Disease: A Critical Review." *Journal of the National Cancer Institute* 22 (1959).

Rabkin, J., and E. L. Struening. "Life Events, Stress, and Illness." *Science,* December 3, 1976, pp. 1013–1020.

Selye, Hans. "The Evolution of the Stress Concept." *American Scientist* 61 (1973), p. 692.

———. *Stress Without Distress*. New York: J. B. Lippincott Company, 1974.

———. *The Stress of Life*. New York: McGraw-Hill Book Company, 1978.

Week Eight: Smoking

Bland, Jeffrey. *Nutraerobics*. San Francisco: Harper & Row, 1983.

Brody, Jane. *Personal Health*. New York: Times Books, 1982.

Saifer, Phyllis, M.D., and Merla Zellerback. *Detox*. Los Angeles: Jeremy P. Tarcher, 1984.

Additional technical medical references have been used in the preparation of this book, the names of which are available from the author.

Index

"Adaptation" energy, 40–41
Addiction(s), 3–5, 6, 35–37, 52–53
  bad habits as, 3–4
  caffeine as, 52–53
  stress as, 35–37
  three signs of, 52
Aerobic dancing, 248
Aerobic fitness, 232, 239–52
  choosing exercises, 245–49
  defined, 240
  F.I.T. formula and, 240–41
  heart rate, how to take, 243
  Modified Step Test, 243–45
  recovery heart rate, 242
  resting heart rate, 241–42
  target heart rate, 242
  See also Exercise
Alcohol, 23, 197–223, 303–04
  accident risks and, 209
  alcoholism, 199
  as appetite diminisher, 213
  "average" consumption of,
    202–03
  awareness of effects of, 220
  benign acceptance of, 198
  biochemical effects of, 208–11

biochemical individuality and,
  203
blood sugar and, 212
brain and nervous system
  affected by, 208–09
caloric value of, 213
cancer and, 211
counting drinks, 221
daily drinking, 219
"drink," defined, 202
driving and, 206, 221–222
as a drug, 205
emotional circumstances and use
  of, 203–04
enhancing pleasure with, 221
enlisting help to give up, 214
"European excuse" and, 204–05
as a food, 205
gastrointestinal system and, 210
glutamine and, 218
immediate effects of, 208
inebriation and, 220
inventory of consumption,
  202–03
limited abstention and, 199
liver and, 211

memory affected by, 209
moderate drinking, 206–08
as most abused substance, 206
nutrition and, 213–14
with other drugs, 210
post-Medical Makeover and, 303–04
problem drinkers, 200–02
psychological addiction, 201–02
"relaxation" drinking, 219–20
resumption of drinking after abstention, 218–22
routines and drinking, 216
saying "no" to, 214–15
sexual performance and, 209–10
situational temptations and, 216–17
stress and, 211–12, 221
substitutes for, 216
three types of consumers of, 197–98
tips on eliminating, 214–17, 219–22, 222–23
vitamin deficiency and, 213
See also Problem drinkers
Alcoholics Anonymous, 199
Alcoholism, 199
indications of, 200
See also Alcohol; Problem drinkers
Allergies:
to vitamins, 195
See also Food allergies
American Chemical Society, 171
American diet, 123–24
chronic diseases and, 123
McGovern committee on, 123
American Health, 91
American Psychiatric Association, 54
Antibiotics, 150–51
Antioxidants, 46, 61
Antistress formula, 46
Antistress hormones, 38, 41–44, 45, 55, 128–29
antistress formula and, 46
body's manufacture of, 45

energy-fatigue cycle and, 42–44
glucose level and, 41
"run-down" state and, 45
Arteriosclerosis, 141, 259
Aspartame, 113

"Balanced diet," 164–67
controlled studies on, 164
"enriched foods" and, 166–67
fresh foods and, 166
processed foods and, 165–66
Ball, Gordon, 134
Balsamic vinegar, 143
Behavioral medicine, 12, 22
Belloc, Nedra, 22
Beltsville Human Nutrition Center, 165
Bennett, Dr. William, 232
Benson, Dr. Herbert, 269–72
relaxation response (RR) of, 269–72
Beta-carotene, 46
Beta-endorphins, 230
"Biochemical boosters," 30, 131–32
chromium, 131
glycemic index, 131
L-tryptophan, 131–32
serotonin levels and, 132
Bioflavinoids, 183–84
Blood sugar, 18, 26, 89, 144, 212, 235, 280, 281, 282
alcohol and, 212
chromium and, 18, 26
smoking and, 279–80, 281, 282
Bran, 145
Breakfast, 96
Breast cancer, 52
Breslow, Lester, 22
Brewer's yeast, 93
Brody, Jane, 284

Caffeine, 29, 49–76, 129, 301–02
addiction to, 50, 52, 62–63
allergy to coffee beans, 69
antioxidants and, 62
biochemical reactions to, 61–62
cancer and, 52

Caffeine (*Cont'd.*)
catecholamines and, 61
coffee advertising and, 52
decaffeinated beverages, 68–69
dieting and, 59–60
diet pills and, 60
diets and, 129
discrimination, tasks involving, 59
effects of, 54–55
elimination of as goal, 50–51, 63
energy and, 57–58
enlisting help in giving up, 73–74
eye-hand coordination and, 59
fatigue and, 57–58
habit *vs.* addiction, 62–63
hand tremors and, 59
headaches and, 55, 74
heart disease and, 53
herbal teas as substitute for, 69–71
high blood pressure and, 53
"high-low cycle" and, 57
hunger attacks and, 60
identifying sources in diet, 64–66
irritations caused by, 55, 74
metabolic half-life of, 55
monitoring elimination of, 75
nicotine and, 56, 73
in over-the-counter drugs, 51
performance and, 58–59
planning elimination campaign, 71
post-Medical Makeover, 301–02
prescription drugs and, 56
products containing (table), 64–66
questions to ask about, 62–63
quitting cold turkey, 67–68
relapses in use of, 76
risks and, 67
sleep and, 56
as socially sanctioned addiction, 52
as stimulant, 54–56
stress and, 61–62
substitute beverages, 69–71
triggers encouraging use of, 71–73
withdrawal symptoms of, 56, 71, 74–75
Caffeinism, 53–54
"anxiety neurosis" and, 53
defined, 53
soft drinks and, 54
Calcium, 86, 162, 186–88
Calisthenics, 249
Cancer, 23, 52, 125, 141, 211
breast, 52
caffeine and, 52
fat and, 141
statistics on, 23
Carbohydrates. *See* Complex carbohydrates
Carbonated beverages, 54, 70
Catecholamines, 61
Chafetz, Dr. Morris, 200
Chemical additives, 149–52
antibiotics, 150–51
common foods containing, 150
diseases and, 150
labels and, 150
sodium nitrate, 151
sodium nitrite, 151
Cholesterol, 124, 141
Chosen illnesses, 21–26
life-style and, 22
medical profession and, 24–26
prevention and, 25
television commercials and, 25
Chromium, 18, 26, 79, 92–94, 99, 131, 189–90, 280
brewer's yeast and, 93
daily requirement, 93
glucose intolerance and, 92
marginal deficiency in, 92
risk of loss, 93
smoking and, 280
sources of, 93
as supplement, 94
Chronic diseases, 10, 36, 124

American diet and, 124
  symptoms of, 35–36
  vague symptoms and, 10
Cigarettes. *See* Smoking
Club soda, 70, 154
Coffee, 6, 7, 23, 68–69
  allergy to beans, 69
  See also Caffeine
Colds, susceptibility to, 10
"Collateral" blood vessels, 234
Complex carbohydrates, 81,
    143–46
  appetite control and, 144
  blood sugar and, 144
  fiber and, 144–45
  increasing amount in diet,
    145–46
  value of, 144
Concentration, 10, 297
Copper, 192–93
Corn syrup, 116
Cross-country skiing, 248
Cycling, 247–48

Dairy products, 141–42
Death rate, 21
Decaffeinated beverages, 68–69
  dangers of, 69
Depression, 10
de Vries, Herbert, 230
Diabetes mellitus, 84–85
*Diagnostic and Statistical Manual
    (III)* (APA), 54
Dieter's Dilemma, The (Bennett
    and Gurin), 232
"Dieter's hypertension," 128
Diethylstilbestrol (DES), 151
Dieting, 59–60, 126–29
  biochemical effects of, 128–29
  caffeine and, 59–60, 129
  as counterproductive, 126–29
  "dieter's hypertension" and, 128
  as negative approach, 126
  stress caused by, 128–29
  time limits on, 127
  weight baseline and, 128
  "yo-yo syndrome," 127

Diet pills, 60
Diet sodas, 116
Disability rate, 21
"Dr. Giller's Tofu Shake," 147–48

Energy-fatigue cycle, 41–43,
    57–58, 88–90
"Enriched foods," 167
Environment Action Bulletin, 151
Epinephrine, 38, 41–44, 55, 128–29
Ernsberger, Paul, 127
"Escape myth," 260–62
Excedrin, 51
Exercise, 224–52, 304
  activity as goal, 226
  aerobic dancing, 248
  aerobic fitness, 232, 239–52
  as antidote, 226–27
  appetite-increase myth, 233
  backlash against, 228–30
  beginning, 236–39
  benefits of, 227–28
  beta-endorphins and, 230
  blood plasma and, 234
  books on, 252
  boredom and, 251
  calisthenics, 249
  calorie burn-up myth, 232
  choosing, 245–49
  "collateral" blood vessels and,
    234
  convenience and, 251
  cross-country skiing, 248
  cycling, 247
  energy levels and, 235
  as enhancement, 227
  enjoying, 249–50
  far-reaching effects of, 225
  with friends, 251–52
  fringe benefits of, 235
  getting started, 252
  HDL and, 234
  heart disease and, 233–35
  importance of, 224–25
  incentive, 230–31
  jogging, 246–47
  maintenance, 249–52

Exercise (Cont'd.)
  medical checkup and, 237
  osteoporosis and, 235
  overenthusiasm for, 238–39
  post-Medical Makeover, 304
  questions to ask about, 236
  regular schedule for, 250
  running, 246–47
  set-point theory of weight and, 232
  smoking and, 234–35
  statistics on, 224–25
  stress test for, 237
  swimming, 248
  three components of fitness, 239
  Type A personality and, 230–31
  walking, 247
  weight and, 231–33
  See also Aerobic fitness.

Fat, 140–43
  cancers and, 141
  heart disease and, 141
  proportion in diet, 140
  steps to reduce amount in diet, 141–43
Fatigue, 4–6, 9, 42–43, 57–58, 136
  and-energy cycle, 42–43, 57–58
Fiber, 144–46
  blood sugar and, 144
  bran, 145
  defined, 145
  increasing amount in diet, 145–46
Fish, 147
F.I.T. formula, 240–41
Folic acid, 181
Food allergies, 135–36
  symptoms, 135–36
  varied diet and, 135
Free radicals, 45
Fried foods, 143
Friedman, Dr. Meyer, 264–65

Glucose, 81–82
Glucose intolerance, 92
Glucose tolerance factor (GTF), 92

Glucose-tolerance test, 87
Glutamine, 218
Glycemic index, 94–96, 131
  chart for carbohydrates, 95–96
  defined, 94
Gurin, Joel, 232

Habits, changing of, 11–15
  addictions, habits as, 4, 16–17
  behavioral medicine and, 12
  biochemically determined habits, 17
  Harris poll and, 15
  health determined by, 12
  inconsistent "rules" and, 13
  motivation and, 14
  techniques for, 16–18
  willpower and, 15–16
HDL (high-density lipoprotein), 234
Headaches, 4, 5, 10, 55–56, 74
  caffeine and, 56, 74
Heart disease, 7, 53, 83–84, 233–35
  caffeine and, 53
  exercise and, 233–35
  sugar and, 83–84
Heckler, Margaret, 144
Herbal teas, 69–71
High blood pressure, 53, 128, 259
  caffeine and, 53
  "dieter's hypertension," 128
Homeostasis, 37–38
Hypertension. See High blood pressure
Hypoallergenic supplements, 195
Hypoglycemia, 84, 86–88, 282

Insulin, 90–91
Iodine, 194
Iron, 163, 193–94
Irritability, 9, 55, 74

Jogging, 246–47

Large meals, 136–37
Late meals, 136
Life-style changes, 11–15

L-tryptophan, 131–32
  carbohydrate cravings and,
    131–32
  dosage, 131
  as sleep inducer, 132

McGovern, George, 123
"Machine theory" of health, 25
Macronutrients, 160
Magnesium, 188–89
Meat, 142
Medical Makeover:
  alcohol (Week Five), 197–223
  "biochemical boosters," 30
  caffeine (Week One), 49–76
  effective sequence of, 29–30
  exercise (Week Six), 224–52
  four steps to using, 32–33
  the future and, 301–07
  habits, changing of, 11–15
  life-style changes, 11–15
  long-term effects, 8
  minerals (Week Four), 172–94
  as new beginning, 305–06
  new confidence and, 306–07
  New Nutrition (Week Three),
    120–55
  origins of, 26–27
  positive medicine and, 21–33
  questions to ask about, 19–20
  reverting to old habits, 299–301
  seven-day-quit-smoking
    program, 287–95
  short-term effects, 8
  smoking (Week Eight), 278–98
  stress and, 34–46
  stress control (Week Seven),
    253–77
  sugar (Week Two), 77–119
  vitamins (Week Four), 156–96
Megavitamin therapy, 159
Minerals, 30, 157, 173–94, 303
  defined, 157
  functions in body, 158
  personal profile, 173–94
  post-Medical Makeover, 303
  See also individual minerals;
    Vitamins

Modified Step Test, 243–45
Motivation, 14–28

"Natural" sugars, 99
New Nutrition, 120–55, 302
  biochemical boosters and, 131–32
  bread and, 153
  changing American diet and,
    123–24
  chemical additives, 149–52
  chronic diseases and, 124
  complex carbohydrates, 143–46
  defined, 124
  diets and, 126–29
  family involvement in, 138–39
  fat and, 141–43
  fiber and, 144–45
  goals of, 121–22, 140
  grocery shopping and, 122,
    139–40, 153
  guidelines for, 125
  large meals, 136–37
  late meals, 136
  leftovers and, 152
  McGovern committee on
    nutrition and, 123
  new eating habits, 132–39
  post-Medical Makeover, 302
  preparation for meals, 137–38
  principles of, 140–52
  protein and, 147–48
  quiz to evaluate habits, 122–23
  regular meals, 133–34
  in restaurants, 153–54
  salt and, 148–49
  sample menu for, 154–55
  shopping lists and, 140
  tips on, 152–55
  varied diet and, 134–36
  weight loss and, 121, 129–31
Niacin. *See* Vitamin B₃
Nicotine, 30, 56, 72. *See also*
  Smoking
Nitrosamine, 283
Norepinephrine, 38, 41–44, 55,
  128–29, 211
Nutrition. *See* New Nutrition
Nutrition quiz, 122–23

Oatmeal, 145
Omega-3 fatty acids, 147
Osteoporosis, 86, 162, 186, 235
Overstimulation, 41–44

Pantothenic acid, 180
Pauling, Linus, 168, 171, 182
    on RDA, 168
    on Vitamin C, 182
Pero, 70
Phosphorus, 86
Pickles, 117
Popcorn, 117
Positive medicine, 21–33
    chosen illnesses, 21–26
    medical profession and, 24–26
    seven basic good health
        practices, 22
    statistics on health, 21
Postum, 70
Poultry, 142
Pritikin, Nathan, 13
Problem drinkers, 200–02, 204,
        206
    defined, 201
    increased tolerance and, 207
    quiz about, 204
Processed foods, 165–66
    "overconsumptive
        undernutrition" and, 166
Protein, 147–48
    meatless meals and, 148
    soy as source of, 147
Proxmire, Sen. William, 168

Recommended Dietary Allowances
        (RDA), 167–70
    conflicts of interest and, 168
    defined, 167
    individuality and, 169–70
    limitations of, 170
Recovery heart rate, 242
Refined carbohydrates, 146
Regular meals (at regular times),
        96–97, 132–34
Relaxation response (RR), 269–72
    benefits of, 270
    method described, 271–72

Resting heart rate, 241–42
Rodin, Dr. Judith, 90
Root vegetables, 146
Rosenman, Dr. Ray, 264–65
Running, 246–47

Saccharin, 113–14
Salads, 146
Salazar, Alberto, 163
Salt, 148–49
Schroeder, Dr. Henry, 165
Sea salt, 149
Selenium, 46, 190–91
Seltzer, 70
Selye, Dr. Hans, 38, 39, 40
Serotonin levels, 132
Seven basic good health practices,
        22
Seven-day-quit-smoking program,
        287–95
Shive, William, 218
Sleep, 132
Smoking (generally), 6, 13, 30,
        · 235, 278–97
    aging and, 283
    diseases and, 283
    exercise and, 234
    hazards of, 282–86
    hypoglycemia and, 282
    nitrosamine and, 283
    pregnancy and, 283
    radiation and, 283
    See also Stopping smoking
Snacks, 96
Sodium nitrate, 151
Sodium nitrite, 151
Soft drinks, 54, 70, 77–78
Stimulants, 54
Stopping smoking, 278–98,
        304–305
    blood sugar levels and, 279–82
    chromium supplement and, 280,
        282
    cold-turkey method, 287
    constipation and, 297
    coughing and, 296
    fatigue and, 296
    metabolic changes, 280–81

post-Medical Makeover, 304–05
seven-day-quit-smoking
  program, 287–95
snacking and, 281
sore throats and, 297
tips from quitters, 297–98
weight gain and, 280–82
withdrawal symptoms, 287,
  295–97
See also Smoking (generally)
Stress, 34–46, 61–62, 88–90,
  127–29
"adaptation" energy, 40
as addiction, 35–37
alcohol and, 211–12
antioxidants and, 46
antistress formula, 46
antistress hormones, 38, 41–44,
  45
appetite stimulants, 42
bad habits and, 35, 41–44
biochemical responses to, 37,
  45
caffeine and, 61–62
chronic diseases and, 35
diets causing, 127–29
energy-and-fatigue cycle, 41–43
epinephrine and, 38, 41–44
"exhaustion stage" of, 39–40
free radicals and, 45
glucose level and, 41–42
homeostasis and, 37–38
long-term effects of, 35–37
norepinephrine and, 38, 41–44
overstimulation and, 41–44
as primitive reaction, 37–38
secret, 44–45
Selye definition of, 38
stress as reaction to, 44–45
sugar and, 88–90
See also Stress control
Stress control, 253–77, 304
active *vs.* passive relaxation, 269
advantages of stress and,
  274–76
behavioral stress symptoms (list),
  267–68
body-relaxation technique,

273–74
buildup of stress and, 262–64
career-oriented people and,
  262–63
"confidence factor" and, 254
diseases and, 259
emotional stress symptoms (list),
  267
"escape myth" and, 260–62
feelings, focus on, 275
high blood pressure and, 259
long-term health and, 260
negative emotions and, 276
physical benefits of, 253–54
post-Medical Makeover, 304
quantifying effects of stress,
  264–66
quiz on stress recognition,
  257–58
relaxation and, 268–72
relaxation response (RR) and,
  269–72
risks of stress, 258–60
tips on, 274–76
triggers and, 272–73
"worst remedies" for stress, 269
See also Stress
Sugar, 26, 30, 70, 77–119, 302
as acceptable addiction, 80, 87
American annual consumption
  of, 77
blood fat level and, 84
blood-sugar fluctuations and, 88
breakfasts and, 97
chromium and, 26, 79, 92–94,
  99
common additives, 100
diabetes mellitus and, 84
diet sodas and, 116
diminishing "sweet tooth" and,
  112
energy-fatigue cycle and, 89–90
enlisting help in giving up,
  118–19
as food additive, 77, 100–01
glucose, 81–82
glycemic index and, 94–96
grocery shopping and, 99

Sugar (cont'd.)
heart disease and, 83–84
"hidden sugar" (chart), 101–10
hypoglycemia and, 84, 86–88
insulin and, 90–91
"natural" sugars, 99
nutritional value of, 82–83
osteoporosis and, 86
post-Medical Makeover and, 302
as preservative, 99
quitting cold turkey, 111–12
quiz on sugar risk, 97–98
reading labels for, 100–10
relapses in use of, 119
snacks and, 97
soft drinks and, 77
starches and, 81–82
step-by-step approach to giving
up, 91–97
stress and, 88–90
substitutes, 112–14
"sugar-free" foods, 101
"sweet tooth" myth, 26
taste for, as anachronism, 81
tips on giving up, 114–19
tooth decay and, 85–86
triggers encouraging use of,
117–18
weight gain and, 90–91
Sugar substitutes, 112–14
aspartame, 113
disadvantages of, 113
saccharin, 113–14
weight control and, 114
"Superficial" energy, 40–41
Supplements:
hypoallergenic, 195
See also Minerals; Vitamins
Sweets, cravings, for, 18, 26
chromium and, 18
myth about, 26
Swimming, 248
Synthetic vitamins, 195

Target heart rate, 242
Television commercials, 24
Tobacco. See Smoking
Tofu, 147–48

"Dr. Giller's Tofu Shake,"
147–48
Tooth decay, 85–86
Triglycerides, 84
Tuna packed in water, 116
Type A Behavior and Your Heart
(Rosenman and Friedman),
264
Type A personality, 230–31

Vague symptoms, 9–11
aging and stress, 9
chronic diseases and, 10–11
ignoring signals, 10
as psychosomatic, 10
Varied diet, 134–36
allergies and, 135
hunger and, 135
nutrition value of, 135
Vitamin A, 173–75
as fat-soluble, 174
Vitamin B₁ (thiamine), 175–76
Vitamin B₂ (riboflavin), 176–78
Vitamin B₃ (niacin), 177–78
Vitamin B₆, 171, 178–79
Vitamin B₁₂, 179–80
Vitamin C, 46, 169, 171, 182–83,
195
Linus Pauling on, 182
Vitamin D, 184–85
Vitamin E, 46, 169, 185–86
as fat-soluble, 185
Vitamin deficiency, 161–63, 213
alcohol and, 213
minor deficiency, signs of, 163
osteoporosis and, 162
three changes and, 162
Vitamins, 30, 156–96, 303
adverse reactions to, 195–96
"balanced diet" and, 164–67
biochemical individuality and,
171–72
confusion about, 158–59, 160–61
deficiency of, 161–63
defined, 157
"enriched foods" and, 166–67
expectations and, 159–60
as facilitators, 160

government tables and, 166
hypoallergenic supplements, 195
megavitamin therapy, 159
personal profile, 173–94
post-Medical Makeover, 303
Recommended Dietary
    Allowance (RDA) and,
    167–70
synthetic *vs.* natural, 195
See also individual vitamins;
    Minerals

Walking, 247
Weight control, 90–91, 129–31,
    231–33, 280–82
exercise and, 231–33
New Nutrition and, 129–31
set-point theory and, 232
smoking and, 280–82
sugar and, 90–91, 129

Weir, Dr. Edith, 166
Whole grains, 145–46
Why You Should Quit Smoking
    (chart), 284–86
Williams, Roger, 171
Willpower, 15–16
Withdrawal symptoms, 56, 74–75,
    287, 295–97
caffeine and, 56, 74–75
smoking and, 287, 295–97
Wurtman, Dr. Judith, 132
Wurtman, Dr. Richard, 131, 132

Yew, Dr. Man-Li, 169
Yogurt, 115, 152
Yudkin, Dr. John, 83

Zinc, 191–92